T0144841

BASIC HEALTH PUBLICATIONS USER'S GUIDE

TO CALCIUM & MAGNESIUM

Learn What You Need to Know about How These Nutrients Build Strong Bones.

NAN KATHRYN FUCHS, PH.D.
JACK CHALLEM Series Editor

The information contained in this book is based upon the research and personal and professional experiences of the author. It is not intended as a substitute for consulting with your physician or other healthcare provider. Any attempt to diagnose and treat an illness should be done under the direction of a healthcare professional.

The publisher does not advocate the use of any particular healthcare protocol but believes the information in this book should be available to the public. The publisher and author are not responsible for any adverse effects or consequences resulting from the use of the suggestions, preparations, or procedures discussed in this book. Should the reader have any questions concerning the appropriateness of any procedures or preparation mentioned, the author and the publisher strongly suggest consulting a professional healthcare advisor.

Series Editor: Jack Challem

Editor: Carol Rosenberg

Typesetter: Gary A. Rosenberg

Series Cover Designer: Mike Stromberg

Basic Health Publications User's Guides are published by Basic Health Publications, Inc.

basichealthpub.com

ISBN-13: 978-1-59120-009-3 (Pbk.)
ISBN-13: 978-1-68162-842-4 (Hardcover)

CONTENTS

INTRODUCTION

Calcium. It's not just a miracle mineral for strong bones. Calcium helps your heart contract, lowers your blood pressure, and nourishes your nerves. In some people, it protects against colon cancer and reduces symptoms of PMS.

But calcium doesn't work alone. Without enough magnesium, calcium can actually cause more harm than good. Calcium is better known than magnesium. But magnesium is so important to our health, and so lacking in our diets, that people who supplement with it often think they've found a miracle mineral. In many ways, they have.

Magnesium is calcium's partner in many body functions. Without enough magnesium, calcium can't get into your bones. It's simply not absorbed. And this unabsorbed calcium can lead to such health problems as arthritis and heart disease. Although a great many supplements contain both calcium and magnesium, you may need more magnesium and less calcium than they contain— especially if you also eat a high-calcium, low-magnesium diet.

A typical American diet tends to be high in calcium and low in magnesium. Most supplements contain more calcium than magnesium, as well. Calcium supplements are among the most widely taken of all nutrients. More people take extra calcium than even vitamin C! The result is that our mineral balance has become calcium heavy and magnesium deficient.

Low magnesium can contribute to high blood pressure, premenstrual mood swings and anxiety, sore muscles, depression, headaches, diabetes, and more. You need plenty of magnesium for a healthy nervous system, for energy, and to build strong bones. When you increase your magnesium, all of these conditions improve. There's no doubt that getting enough calcium is extremely important. But getting adequate magnesium is often even more important.

If you're taking a lot of calcium and not paying attention to magnesium, it's probably because that's the advice you've heard. It's information that's generally accepted as being accurate. However, the amount of calcium and magnesium you've been told to take is based on very old research. Newer studies indicate that we need less calcium and more magnesium than previously thought.

This *User's Guide to Calcium & Magnesium* is designed to clear up the confusion about these two very important minerals and explain how they work together. It will answer your questions about the role of calcium and magnesium in various diseases and help you decide how much of each you need to get and stay healthy.

Each of our bodies has slightly different needs so not everyone needs the same amount of every nutrient. This is not a "one size fits all" situation. There are always variables that are not addressed in the studies that have been conducted. Your body's calcium and magnesium requirements may not only be different from someone else's, they may also change with age, stress, the medications you take, and your particular health conditions.

The amount of calcium and magnesium you

need depends also on their forms. Not all of the minerals we get in our food or supplements can be well absorbed. Some forms of calcium and magnesium are well absorbed, like calcium citrate and magnesium citrate-malate. Others are not, like calcium carbonate and magnesium oxide. Since unabsorbed calcium can cause painful and life-threatening health problems, it's important to understand which forms are best absorbed and to use only them.

This guide helps you understand how your particular health and age affect your body's needs for calcium and magnesium. With this information, you can decide how much of each of these important minerals your body needs, and in which forms.

CHAPTER 1

UNDERSTANDING CALCIUM

You can't escape it. News about calcium is everywhere—in magazines, on TV, and in newspapers. Everybody's talking about the need for extra calcium to prevent osteoporosis. The reason for this is that 98 percent of all calcium is needed to continuously make bone. But if you think that calcium's only job is to build strong bones, you're mistaken. Calcium is essential for heart and nerve function, even though only 2 percent gets used for that purpose.

The 2 percent of calcium that stays in your blood and soft tissues is vitally important to your health and well-being. All of your muscles—including your heart—need calcium to contract. In addition, your blood needs calcium to clot. And your nervous system needs enough calcium to send messages throughout your body.

The problem is that you may be taking too much of a good thing. Taking too much calcium can be as much of a problem as getting too little. Excessive amounts of calcium can contribute to muscle cramping, heart palpitations and heart disease, fibromyalgia (nonspecific muscle pain), and some premenstrual syndrome (PMS) symptoms.

This is why it's important to take the amount of calcium your particu-

Cofactor
A substance that helps another substance perform its functions.

lar body needs, and to take it in an easy-to-absorb form. Since calcium doesn't work alone, it's essential to take it with enough of its cofactors. Calcium can't be well absorbed or be used effectively without other nutrients, such as vitamin D, potassium, iron, and magnesium.

Why Calcium Is So Important

Calcium is the most abundant mineral in your body. Almost all of it is in your bones. Don't think of bones as being dead sticks that hold your body together and keep you from collapsing. They are living tissues that are constantly breaking down and being rebuilt. The minerals that make up bone tissue need to be constantly available so that bone can be made continuously. Since some calcium is naturally excreted from your body every day, you need to get sufficient calcium in your diet and supplements every day.

In addition, your body needs calcium to help transmit nerve impulses along nerve cells to send messages across your nervous system. Calcium also helps blood to clot and is involved in many other chemical reactions throughout your body.

One of calcium's major jobs is to help all of the muscles in your body to contract. Magnesium, on the other hand, helps them to relax. Together, these minerals regulate your heartbeat by contracting and relaxing as necessary. So, calcium is vital to a healthy heart. The right amount of calcium helps maintain a regular heartbeat, but too much or too little calcium can cause an irregular heartbeat, called an arrhythmia.

What do minerals do?
Minerals help build bones and connective tissues. They also help messages travel along the nerves and support enzyme production.

Because too much calcium can contribute to health problems, it's important to take just the right amount. This can be confusing because different people look at the amount of calcium we need differently.

RDAs, DRIs, and Other Opinions

There are a lot of opinions about how much calcium we need. Most medical doctors and registered dieticians follow the recommended guidelines given by a government agency. The Food and Nutrition Board of the National Academy of Sciences/National Research Council has assessed our need for nutrient doses at various stages of our lives based on a number of studies. This government agency updates the recommended amount of vitamins and minerals as new information becomes available.

Recommended Daily Allowances (RDA)
Recommendations for the amount of nutrients an "average" healthy person's body needs.

However, there are always conflicting studies giving different information. The amount of any nutrient this government agency says we need is called either an RDA or a DRI.

Dietary Reference Intakes (DRI)
A combination of RDAs and other values. Presently, they're essentially the same as RDAs and may be used interchangeably.

The RDAs for calcium for adolescents and adults are between 1,000 and 1,300 mg a day.

- Males and females ages 25 to 49: 1,000 mg per day.
- Males and females over age 50: 1,200 mg per day.
- Adolescents and teens: 1,300 mg per day.
- Children ages 4 to 8: 800 mg per day.
- Pregnant and lactating women: 1,000 mg per day.

Grams and Milligrams

A gram (g) is a unit of weight. One pound equals 454 grams. A milligram (mg) is one-thousandth of a gram.

Even though these recommended amounts are based on scientific studies, numerous doctors, scientists, and nutritionists are finding that these doses don't work for all of their patients. If only it was this simple, all we would need to do is to find the RDA or DRI for calcium and take that amount. Unfortunately, it's not that cut-and-dried. Not only are many health practitioners questioning the RDA for calcium, newer studies are finding that these amounts may be too high for many people, especially if they already have health problems.

Many health practitioners are finding that 500 mg of supplemental calcium a day reduces health conditions like heart disease and fibromyalgia, and still protects bone density. If you look only at RDAs and DRIs without considering your body's individual needs, you may be overlooking important information that could impact your health greatly.

These RDAs and DRIs are based on the amount of calcium a healthy person needs, but these standards do not account for individual differences in absorption. People with serious health conditions like colon cancer and heart disease need more or less calcium. Also, many people are neither sick nor healthy, but are somewhere in between. They can have symptoms of a calcium deficiency or excess, but these symptoms may not be severe enough to be called a particular disease. To meet your particular calcium requirements, you need to look more closely at your age, health, and diet.

Calcium for Osteoporosis

The most popular reason for taking large amounts of calcium is to prevent osteoporosis. Fear motivates many women to take more than their bodies can use. Wherever we turn, we see advertisements for calcium supplements that show women's bodies bent and twisted from osteoporosis. These ads are designed to help sell more calcium supplements. And they do. In theory, taking a lot of calcium may make sense. But in practice, it doesn't always work. In fact, it can backfire.

To prevent osteoporosis, calcium has to get absorbed into your bones. David Levinson, M.D., of the Cornell University Medical Center in New York City, found that the highest amount of calcium anyone should take at one time for good absorption is just 500 mg. This makes sense. If you look at the amount of calcium in many healthy meals, it rarely tops 500 mg. Over the centuries, our bodies have learned to utilize that amount at any one time, but not a great deal more.

Absorption
The passage of substances, such as the nutrients in food, into the blood and tissues.

It's not unusual for people to take 1,000–1,500 mg of calcium supplements a day in addition to any calcium in the foods they eat. And they often take these supplements all at once, so they won't forget to take them later. The problem is that very little of these high amounts of calcium can be absorbed. Perhaps this is one reason why an article published in *The New England Journal of Medicine* reported that a two-year clinical study that gave 2,000 mg of calcium a day showed little to no effect on bone density in its participants.

Other studies have had similar findings. A four-year Mayo Clinic study, also published in *The New England Journal of Medicine*, divided its participants into two groups. One group took 1,400 mg of calcium supplements a day. The other group took less than 500 mg. The rate of bone loss in both groups was the same. Clearly, there's more to bone density than taking a lot of calcium.

Osteoporosis
A condition of reduced bone density and increased bone brittleness that can lead to bones that break easily. More bone flexibility, or increased bone density, reduces fracture rates.

When you take more calcium than you can use, the extra calcium isn't automatically excreted. In fact, it can contribute to uncomfortable and dangerous conditions like arthritis and heart disease. The key is to take the right amount of a well-absorbed form of calcium along with other nutrients needed to help it work.

Make Sure Your Body Can Use Calcium

Calcium doesn't work alone. In order to perform various functions, it requires cofactors like magnesium and phosphorus, along with vitamins A, B_6, C, D, and E. Of all the cofactors calcium needs, magnesium is perhaps the most important. It helps carry calcium into the bones, and it allows muscles to relax, after calcium causes them to contract.

Dairy products are high in calcium, but they don't have enough magnesium to help move it into your bones. Whole grains and green leafy vegetables, on the other hand, contain calcium as well as many of its cofactors. A combination of a little dairy along with some whole grains and green vegetables may be your best approach to getting sufficient calcium in your food. However, dairy is not essential. Even vegans can get plenty of calcium if they eat a healthy diet.

Vegan
A vegetarian who does not eat eggs or dairy. Vegans can get enough calcium if their diets contain sufficient servings of beans, whole grains, nuts, and green vegetables.

Before your body can use calcium, it has to be absorbed. Some calcium supplements are poorly absorbed; others are better absorbed. Calcium seems to be best absorbed when it is in the presence of some kind of acid. This acid may be in your food, or it may be the acid secreted by your stomach to help with digestion. The form of calcium you take helps determine how much of this mineral gets into your body. Calcium carbonate, for example, is low in acid and is very poorly absorbed by people who have low stomach acid compared with the more acidic calcium citrate. (More about this later.)

How Age Affects Your Need for Calcium

You have a smart body. It knows which nutrients you need and how to conserve them. It knows that the need for calcium is highest in pregnant women, babies, young children, and young adults, when most bone tissue is forming.

Teens need a lot of calcium. This is because the teen years are the body's last chance to store away extra calcium in the bones and protect them against bone loss later in life. So at these times when we need the most calcium, our bodies absorb it best and excrete it less.

A baby whose bones are forming rapidly can absorb up to 400 mg of calcium a day and excretes only 10 to 40 mg. Calcium absorption changes dramatically after age twenty. From then on, our bodies excrete more calcium and retain less than before—except during pregnancy. An adult absorbs only 20 to 30 percent of the calcium they consume. Postmenopausal women can often absorb no more than 7 percent. While some might interpret this to mean that postmenopausal women should be taking very high amounts of calcium, remember that whatever the body doesn't absorb and excrete can create other health problems.

Adults don't excrete all the unused calcium in their diets and supplements. This is why it's so important for all adults to make certain that the calcium they take is absorbed as well as possible. If your body can't absorb and store it as well as when you were younger, your choice of calcium sources becomes extremely important.

You need about the same amount of calcium as an older adult as you needed as a younger adult. It's just that as you age, less calcium gets absorbed and more is excreted. Again, it's not only the amount of calcium you take that's important with aging, but also calcium absorption and retention.

Other factors enter the calcium-absorption picture as you get older. Poor kidney function can affect calcium absorption. To prevent too much calcium from being excreted in your urine, your kidneys save and reuse some of it. If your kidneys are not working properly, they may not be conserving enough calcium. When this happens, calcium gets stored in soft tissues rather than in bones. This can lead to arthritis, heart disease, hypertension, and even senile dementia.

Digestion and Calcium Absorption

Poor digestion can greatly affect your calcium absorption because of the connection between calcium absorption and acid. A number of studies suggest that calcium needs some form of acid in order to be broken down into a useable form. If you don't have enough acid present with calcium, you may not be absorbing it well. While not all studies have come to this conclusion, your calcium absorption should increase if you take it with some form of acid.

Fortunately, your smart body already makes an acid. When you eat, your stomach secretes hydrochloric acid (HCl). This acid helps digest protein. It also helps break down calcium, magnesium, and other minerals. But as we get older, our bodies make less HCl.

When you chew your food, a message travels from your taste buds to your stomach, telling it to secrete HCl. One method of increasing calcium absorption is simply to chew your food better. This can help your digestion in general, as well as increase your body's ability to use calcium.

Antacids have the opposite effect. They interfere with calcium absorption. Antacids neutralize HCl, reducing that very same acid that helps your body break down and use calcium. If you don't have much HCl due to aging, or if you're taking antacids, there's another possible solution (unless you're unable to eat the following suggested foods and beverages). You can accompany foods high in calcium with small amounts of tomato, orange juice, lemon water, or a little vinegar. The acids in these foods and beverages can help break down and utilize calcium. For instance, when you add an oil-and-vinegar dressing to a salad, you absorb more of the calcium in the salad greens, as well as the calcium in any cheese that may be contained in either the salad or dressing.

Antacid
Something that neutralizes hydrochloric acid (HCl), the acid produced in the stomach. Aluminum hydroxide is one agent that acts as an antacid.

The connection between calcium and HCl is not clear-cut. Robert R. Recker, M.D., is one of several authors of a study published in the journal *Calcified Tissue International.* This study found that HCl is needed to break down calcium, but it wasn't essential for calcium absorption. In a previous study, however, Dr. Recker found that people with low HCl had poor calcium absorption.

Since we don't know exactly what role acid plays in the utilization of calcium, you may want to take steps to maximize calcium absorption. First, take calcium supplements with your meals. Avoid antacids whenever possible. Take calcium with acidic foods. And chew all your food better to help your body secrete needed HCl.

Antacids and Calcium Absorption

Many doctors insist that antacids are a perfectly good source of calcium supplementation because they are inexpensive and high in calcium. If your doctor recommends that you take calcium-containing antacids instead of another form of calcium, ask why. Acid helps the body utilize calcium.

Numerous studies have concluded that antacids are not protective against osteoporosis. A six-year study of more than 6,000 women, published in the *New England Journal of Medicine*, found that women who used Tums antacid as their only source of supplemental calcium had more broken arms than women who didn't. This was a large enough study to get the attention of many people, but not enough to stop doctors from suggesting their patients continue to use this inexpensive form of calcium.

Another study of more than 9,000 women over age sixty-five studied calcium intake versus broken bones. Information on broken bones was collected every four months for more than six years. Those women who took high-calcium antacids had more broken arms than those who took other forms of calcium.

The calcium in antacids is calcium carbonate, a poorly absorbed form of calcium that needs to be in the presence of some kind of acid before your body can use it. The calcium in an antacid begins by being difficult to absorb. Then, if you take an antacid with a high-calcium meal, you will not be able to absorb much of the calcium in your food, either. Antacids may prevent heartburn, but the calcium they contain isn't your best source of absorbable calcium.

What about Prilosec or other drugs that block the production of HCl? They may also interfere with calcium absorption. However, if you have an ulcer, acid reflux, or other medical condition where HCl causes pain, you may need to continue taking these medications, even if they affect your calcium levels.

The Consequences of Too Much Calcium

If you're boosting your calcium intake both in your diet and in supplements just to be on the safe side—take another look at what you're doing. This approach is not necessarily safe, and it could even be dangerous. Extra calcium can cause as many problems as not having enough. And taking a lot of calcium doesn't guarantee that it's getting into your bones.

Guy E. Abraham, M.D., is a research gynecologist and endocrinologist who has researched the subject of calcium and magnesium for decades. He has also published dozens of studies in scientific journals. Dr. Abraham points out that when calcium isn't absorbed into your bones, it doesn't just magically disappear. It can lead to clogged arteries (atherosclerosis). Or it can collect in your joints where it contributes to arthritis, or in your kidneys where it can contribute to the formation of kidney stones.

In addition to clogging your arteries, calcium can accumulate in your aorta. This can reduce the aorta's elasticity and lead to heart disease. When too much calcium gets into muscle tissues, it can produce muscle cramps and fibromyalgia (nonspecific muscle pain). Excessive calcium can also cause irritability, while the right amount can keep you calm.

Stephen Seely, a professor of cardiology in England, wrote in the *International Journal of Cardiology* that many diseases could be avoided if calcium consumption was reduced. He found that hypertension in older age is virtually nonexistent in countries where calcium intake is low.

Too much calcium doesn't protect your bones. In fact, it can lead to the formation of brittle bones that break easily. To avoid this brittleness, you need to be getting plenty of magnesium in your diet and supplements. Magnesium makes bones more flexible and less prone to breaking. Some nutrients strengthen bones, while others, surprisingly, have the opposite effect.

Calcium, Vitamin C, and Broken Hips

You'd think that it's a good idea to take a lot of vitamin C and calcium. Many people do. But it may not be a good idea or even safe. Here's an example of when "more" may not be "better." It concerns women who take a lot of vitamin C along with high amounts of calcium. A Swedish study with 65,000 participants published in the *International Journal of Epidemiology* found that women who took high amounts of both vitamin C and calcium had the highest number of hip fractures. When they reduced their vitamin C intake, they had fewer cases of broken hips.

We don't know what would have happened if they reduced their intake of calcium and not vitamin C. But it seems clear that the combination may not be as beneficial as you thought. For now, you may want to take high quantities of vitamin C supplements as needed, and just the amount of calcium your body needs.

Take a Look at the Whole Picture

It should be clear by now that calcium doesn't work alone, that too much calcium can cause health problems, and that high amounts of calcium are not the answer to forming and maintaining healthy bones. So what's next?

First, take a closer look at magnesium, a mineral you may know little about. Once you understand what magnesium does, you'll be ready to take a look at various health conditions and the role of both calcium and magnesium in each. From there, you can decide how much calcium you need, and how much magnesium should accompany it.

CHAPTER 2

UNDERSTANDING MAGNESIUM

Magnesium is at least as important as calcium. It not only affects the health of your bones, it also plays a significant role in a wide number of body functions. You need lots of magnesium for strong bones, a healthy heart, and to alleviate PMS (premenstrual syndrome) and muscle cramps.

While most calcium is stored in bones, most magnesium remains in your muscles. Calcium causes muscles to contract, while magnesium helps them to relax. Your heart is a muscle that relies on this combination of relaxing and contracting. All of your muscles contain, and need, more magnesium than calcium. It is extremely important that you get enough magnesium for all muscle-related conditions including arrhythmia (irregular heartbeat), headaches, muscle cramps, fibromyalgia, and restless leg syndrome.

But magnesium does even more. It is a natural, safe calcium-channel blocker, protecting you against heart disease. And it is just as important as calcium in preventing osteoporosis. In addition, magnesium helps reduces stress by having a calming effect.

Magnesium's Many Functions

Magnesium works both in partnership with calcium, and independently. On its own, magnesium helps "turn on" hundreds of enzymes. These enzymes allow the carbohydrates (starches and sugars) and fats in your diet to be used as energy. So getting enough magnesium is important in fighting fatigue.

Calcium-Channel Blocker
A substance, often a drug, that protects against heart disease by preventing excess calcium from getting into the smooth muscles of your heart.

Magnesium also helps regulate nerve cell function, allowing your nervous system to relax. One sign of stress that can signal a need for more magnesium is a sensitivity to loud noises.

Magnesium helps your mood and affects how well you sleep. Serotonin is a chemical that produces a feeling of well-being. Melatonin is a hormone that helps you sleep. You can't produce enough of either of these brain chemicals without sufficient magnesium.

Melatonin
A hormone made from serotonin that helps regulate hormone secretion, sleepiness, and wakefulness. Supplemental melatonin can help prevent jet lag.

Our bodies make less and less melatonin as we age. In addition, many older people eat diets low in magnesium, which could boost their melatonin production. If you're depressed or have trouble sleeping, you may not need an antidepressant or a sleeping pill. You may just need more magnesium.

Magnesium and Calcium Work Together

You want your heart muscle to both contract and relax. Because calcium causes your muscles to contract while magnesium helps them to relax, you need a balance of these two minerals for a healthy heart. If you have too many contractions and not enough relaxing, you can have an irregular heartbeat or a heart attack.

Magnesium can prevent and reverse constipation. Your colon is a long muscle that requires calcium and magnesium to contract and relax, allowing waste products to be eliminated. If you have too much calcium or not enough magnesium, you may have spasms in your colon. Or you could become constipated. After ruling out more serious problems, many health practitioners now look at constipation as a possible sign of a magnesium deficiency.

RDAs for Magnesium

Of all the RDAs, the ones for magnesium may be the most misleading. With diets already low in magnesium, and increased magnesium excretion from stress and other health conditions, your need for this mineral may be greater than the RDAs suggest. Author and physician Alan R. Gaby, M.D., is just one of a growing number of medical doctors with a practice that focuses on nutrition. He has found that most of his patients are magnesium-deficient.

The RDAs for magnesium are between 320 and 420 mg a day for adolescents and adults. Interestingly, although there are more signs of magnesium deficiency symptoms in women than in men, magnesium RDAs are higher for men than for women.

- Males ages 25 to 49: 420 mg per day.

- Females ages 25 to 49: 320 mg per day.

- Children ages 4 to 8: 130 mg per day.

- Pregnant and lactating women: 310–360 mg per day.

How to Know If You Need More Magnesium

If your diet is low in magnesium-rich foods like whole grains, nuts, seeds, and beans, chances are you need more magnesium. This is especially true if you eat a lot of dairy products, which are high in calcium with almost no magnesium.

Most dietary supplements contain twice as much calcium as magnesium. In theory, this may reflect the body's need for these two minerals. But practically speaking, years of stress and diets low in magnesium upset nature's balance. Many people need at least as much magnesium as calcium. If you take high calcium supplements with half as much magnesium, or less, chances are you would benefit from more magnesium.

Are you a chocoholic? It may be a sign that you have a magnesium deficiency. Chocolate is very high in magnesium. If you crave chocolate, either all the time or when you are premenstrual and your need for magnesium increases, you may need more magnesium. Constipation, irregular heartbeat, muscle cramps, and muscle pain (fibromyalgia) are all signs of a possible need for more magnesium.

Why So Many People Are Low in Magnesium

Blame it on your ancestors. Research gynecologist and endocrinologist Guy E. Abraham, M.D., looked back in history and found an interesting explanation for magnesium deficiencies. Thousands of years ago, he discovered, our ancestors ate diets high in magnesium—nuts, seeds, whole grains, and beans. In fact, the magnesium in their diets often provided them with twice as much magnesium as calcium. Dairy products were not abundant at that time, so their calcium intake was low.

Their bodies adapted to this low-calcium, high-magnesium diet by retaining and reusing calcium. Since magnesium was available on a daily basis, unused magnesium was excreted. Our bodies still function like those of our ancestors. Our kidneys still recycle some calcium, but don't retain magnesium. This is why we need to concentrate on getting enough magnesium every day.

Both calcium and magnesium are important. But Dr. Abraham is one of a growing number of health practitioners who has found that getting enough magnesium corrects a wide number of health problems. Unfortunately, you can't just get a blood test to see if you're getting enough magnesium.

The Problem with Magnesium Blood Tests

They're just not accurate, says Mildred S. Seelig, M.D., one of the world's authorities on magnesium. Magnesium is a difficult mineral to measure. When you have a yearly blood test, you can have your magnesium level tested. But this test, called serum magnesium, may not reveal low magnesium.

Some doctors, including Dr. Abraham, believe that a Red Blood Cell (RBC) magnesium test is a better indicator of magnesium levels. But not all laboratories do this particular test, and many doctors are unfamiliar with it. Studies have shown that there are no blood tests that are sensitive enough to accurately diagnose magnesium deficiencies.

So where does this leave you? Dr. Seelig suggests that taking more magnesium than the RDAs is safe unless you have kidney problems. The primary common side effect from taking too much magnesium is loose bowels. There's an easy way to tell whether or not you have a magnesium deficiency. Increase your magnesium for a few months and see if your symptoms lessen or disappear.

Some Symptoms of Low Magnesium

Sherry Rogers, M.D., of Syracuse, New York, finds

that one of the most common symptoms of magnesium deficiency is pain in the back or neck. But there are many other signs as well.

Low magnesium can cause high blood pressure, irritability, nervousness, and anxiety. It can lead to muscle cramps and spasms and muscle tension, including constipation. Magnesium deficiency can cause depression, fatigue, exhaustion, learning disabilities, and an excessive sensitivity to noise and pain. If that wasn't enough, it can contribute to poor appetite—even anorexia—and irregular or rapid heartbeat.

Problems from Taking Too Much Magnesium

You can take too much of a good thing, even when it's magnesium. But for the most part, magnesium is a very safe nutrient to increase due to its self-limiting attributes. When you take more magnesium than your body can handle, you're likely to have intestinal gas or loose stools.

Some doctors suggest you take magnesium "to bowel tolerance." This means taking enough to allow you to have stools that are comfortable, but not too loose. Some practitioners begin by adding 100 mg of magnesium a day for a few days. If their patients' stools aren't too soft, they increase it gradually until the stools are comfortably soft.

If your stools are already soft and you suspect a magnesium deficiency, you have a few choices. Begin by increasing your dietary magnesium: whole grains, nuts, seeds, beans, and dark green vegetables. Then try taking magnesium glycinate, a form of magnesium that is less likely to cause loose bowels. If you can't find magnesium glycinate, try magnesium from amino acid chelate. It works almost as well.

Finally, if your need for magnesium still seems

clear, talk with your doctor about a more extreme, but effective solution: getting magnesium injections. Before you do, however, make sure that your body is able to use the magnesium you're already taking.

Absorbing and Using Magnesium

If you can't absorb magnesium, your body can't use it. Several dietary factors get in the way of magnesium absorption and utilization. Both a high-fat diet and a diet high in phosphorus block magnesium absorption. So begin by looking at your diet to see if you're unknowingly getting in your own way and creating a magnesium deficiency.

The phosphoric acid in most cola drinks, along with the phosphates in baking powder, processed meats and cheeses, and other processed foods, combines with magnesium to form a substance called magnesium phosphate. The majority of the magnesium you take is able to be absorbed in your intestines. But magnesium phosphate prevents magnesium from being absorbed and causes it to be excreted in solid wastes.

A high-fat diet also reduces the availability of magnesium. When fats combine with magnesium, they turn into a soapy consistency that can't get into your intestines and become absorbed. Diets high in fried foods, cheese, and fatty meats all interfere with your body's ability to use magnesium.

Perhaps the least known reason for poor magnesium absorption is getting too much calcium either in your diet or in supplements. Because both calcium and magnesium are absorbed through the same parts of your intestines, when you have too much calcium, you block magnesium absorption.

The amount of available magnesium that is able to keep you healthy depends on how much you take, how much is absorbed, and how much is excreted. Some factors cause your body to excrete more magnesium than it should.

Excessive Magnesium Loss

Your body loses magnesium from diarrhea, diet, and stress. Diarrhea causes much of the magnesium in your intestines to be excreted. The diarrhea may be a result of illness or laxative abuse. It doesn't matter. The results are the same. Some of the foods you eat and the supplements you take also cause increased magnesium excretion.

Magnesium excretion is promoted by drinking too much alcohol or caffeine and by eating high amounts of animal protein or sugar. The kind of sugar that contributes to low magnesium is not limited to refined sugar. It includes fructose, the sugar found in fruits and fruit juices. To prevent too much magnesium from being excreted unnecessarily, reduce your intake of these foods and beverages.

All kinds of stress contribute to excessive magnesium loss. The reason for this is simple. Your adrenal glands make hormones that allow you to handle stressful situations. When these hormone levels get too high, magnesium spills out in the urine. Stress does not just mean a difficult emotional time. It includes mental, physical, thermal (being too hot or too cold), and other kinds of stress. Very loud noises, like fireworks or music played at many rock concerts, can cause this stress response and contribute to magnesium excretion, as well.

Adrenal Glands
These glands, which sit on top of your kidneys, make hormones in response to stress that provide increased energy for emergencies. Due to overstimulation, many people today suffer from adrenal exhaustion and low magnesium.

How Magnesium Influences Calcium Absorption

Calcium absorption is governed by the parathyroid gland, a tiny gland that sits behind the thyroid (a gland in your neck). But magnesium is part of the equation. Your body can't use the calcium in either your diet or supplements without enough magnesium. Here's how it works.

Parathyroid Gland
A small gland that secretes hormones used to regulate calcium and phosphorus metabolism.

Your parathyroid makes hormones called PTH (parathyroid hormones). PTH controls calcium absorption. But your parathyroid needs enough magnesium to make sufficient PTH for calcium absorption.

An interesting study in the *American Journal of Clinical Medicine* reported that taking one gram (1,000 mg) of magnesium a day increases the absorption of *both* calcium and magnesium. When you take extra magnesium, your calcium levels can go up even higher than your magnesium levels. If you're concerned about getting enough useable calcium, you have to first get enough magnesium.

Evaluate Your Mineral Needs

The amount of calcium and magnesium you need depends to a great extent on a number of factors that differ from person to person. You may be someone who can take the RDA of each and be fine. But to best use these minerals to support your health, it's a good idea to look more closely at each condition that is dependent on both calcium and magnesium, and evaluate your body's particular needs.

In the following chapters, you will find information on calcium and magnesium that can help reduce your risk for heart disease, osteoporosis, headaches, muscle cramps, fibromyalgia, and PMS.

You will find out how to use these minerals to support your body during pregnancy, and how they can help improve your mood and energy. Used properly, calcium and magnesium can both prevent health disorders and often reverse them.

CHAPTER 3

PROTECTING YOUR HEART

A healthy heart needs both calcium and magnesium in the right amounts and balance to help it beat regularly and to keep your blood pressure regulated and stable. Magnesium is nature's calcium-channel blocker. It prevents extra calcium that your body can't use from damaging your heart cells. It keeps calcium from clogging up and hardening your arteries. So getting enough magnesium is key to having a healthy heart.

On the other hand, some people with high blood pressure need more calcium than they're getting. So the balance between these two minerals is very important. This is why you need to look at your present health and your family's health history to help evaluate just how much of each you need.

How Calcium and Magnesium Regulate Your Heart

Your heart is a muscle that pumps by constantly contracting and relaxing. Calcium helps your heart and other muscles to contract. Magnesium helps them to relax. Together, they work as a team to keep your heart pumping day and night.

Both of these minerals also help send electrical messages to your heart, reminding it to contract regularly. Too much of either one can lead to heart problems by upsetting a delicate balance.

Magnesium also dilates (opens up) blood vessels in your heart, arms, and legs. This allows more oxygen to flow to your heart. Minerals researcher Thomas Steinmetz found that a magnesium deficiency was the cause of death from sudden heart attacks in 8 million people in this country between 1940 and 1994. Clearly, magnesium is not only important to a healthy heart function. It is also essential in preventing heart problems.

Calcium-Channel Blockers

Calcium that's not absorbed into your bones or other tissues can collect in your arteries where it can lead to atherosclerosis. When this buildup reduces the amount of blood from flowing through your arteries, you can have a heart attack.

Atherosclerosis
A type of hardening of the arteries caused by deposits of either cholesterol or unused calcium.

The idea is to prevent calcium from building up in your arteries. This calls for something to block calcium deposits—a calcium-channel blocker. A number of pharmaceutical drugs are calcium-channel blockers. Magnesium is a natural substance that has the same effect. You can use magnesium, drugs, or both to prevent excess calcium from clogging your arteries.

Procardia and Cardizem are two medications commonly prescribed to block calcium deposits and to regulate heart arrhythmias. All drugs have side effects in some people, and calcium-channel blocking drugs are no exception. Magnesium has the same blocking activity and also regulates the heartbeat with no side effect except, occasionally, loose stools. And magnesium does more than just block calcium deposits and help regulate your heartbeat. It opens up your arteries to allow more blood to flow through, as well.

Don't think you can just stop taking your medications and use magnesium instead. You may be able to, but this is a decision that should be made with your doctor's input and with your being monitored. If you think additional magnesium could be helpful to your heart, talk with your doctor first—especially if you have a heart condition or are at risk for heart disease. If magnesium is a viable option, you may find that when you increase your magnesium you don't need to take calcium-channel blocking drugs. Some people use both magnesium and medications. Be sure to check this out with your doctor before making any changes.

Magnesium's Role in Heart Disease

Low magnesium has been seen in people with irregular or rapid heartbeat, and mitral valve prolapse, a disorder of the heart valves. Magnesium is also often low in people with congestive heart failure and high blood pressure.

A review of magnesium and the heart in *The American Journal of Medicine* found that low magnesium is so common that as many as 65 percent of patients in intensive care suffer from it. What's interesting about this finding is that these low magnesium levels were determined through blood tests. That's right. The same inaccurate blood tests that frequently miss detecting low magnesium in many people. If 65 percent of this group of people were found to have low magnesium using inaccurate tests, it's likely that more accurate tests would reveal a still greater need for additional magnesium.

Surviving a Heart Attack

Magnesium can save your life if you're having a heart attack. If you or anyone you are with is having a heart attack, call 911 and ask the paramedics or emergency room doctor to administer a magnesium IV immediately. Emergency room doctors around the country are now giving intravenous magnesium to people who have heart attacks or heart spasms because it helps reduce mortality.

One study of more than a hundred heart attack patients found that the survival rate increased almost ten times when patients were given additional magnesium. In a review of heart attacks and magnesium published in the journal *Circulation,* intravenous magnesium was given to 1,300 patients. There was a significant reduction in their irregular heartbeats and death.

It's worth discussing the subject of using magnesium for heart attacks with your doctor. Have this information added to your chart so that if it is ever necessary, you and your doctor will know your desire to be given additional magnesium.

Calcium and Arrhythmias

When your blood test shows high serum calcium, you're at an increased risk for irregular heartbeats, or arrhythmias. Irregular heartbeats can lead to blood clots and stroke.

Melvyn R. Werbach, M.D., explains that even when your blood magnesium level is normal, you may be able to reduce your irregular heartbeat by taking more magnesium. He also found that when magnesium is known to be low, it may be necessary to take higher than normal amounts of magnesium supplements to eliminate arrhythmias.

Calcium's Role in a Healthy Heart

Your heart needs calcium, but not too much of it. High amounts of calcium can be harmful, especially if you don't have enough magnesium to use it. But you do need enough calcium for your heart to keep contracting regularly.

As you age, a number of factors can lead to heart problems. These include getting less calcium, making less stomach acid (hydrochloric acid, or HCl), getting less vitamin D (the sunshine vitamin), and having poor calcium absorption through your intestines.

Since your heart can't function without enough calcium, if you're not getting enough in your diet and supplements to help it contract, your body will pull calcium out of your bones. This can lead to osteoporosis, or brittle bones. So for a healthy heart and strong bones, you may want to consider getting equal amounts of calcium and magnesium.

Regulating Your Blood Pressure

If you have high blood pressure (hypertension), you may need more calcium—or more magnesium. Some people need more of one; others need more of the other.

Many people with high blood pressure have diets low in calcium. They may need more calcium to reduce their blood pressure. A study in *The New England Journal of Medicine* reported that group of people with high blood pressure were given 1,000 mg of calcium a day for four months. At the end of that time, their blood pressure was reduced significantly. David A. McCarron, M.D., also found that calcium lowered blood pressure. He noticed that when people were hypertensive (had high blood pressure), they excreted more calcium in their urine than necessary. When he added calcium to their diets, their blood pressure began to drop.

Diuretic Something that increases the excretion of urine. Diuretics may be either herbal or pharmaceutical.

But sometimes it takes more magnesium to lower blood pressure. Nutritionist Ann Louise Gittleman, M.S., C.N.S., found that some people with high blood pressure, especially those taking diuretics, have low magnesium levels. Diuretics not only lower potassium, they also cause more magnesium than usual to be excreted in the urine.

A need for magnesium to lower blood pressure is not limited to people using diuretics. A study published in the *British Medical Journal* found that nineteen out of twenty people lowered their high blood pressure using magnesium supplements. No one in the control group experienced that effect.

If you have high blood pressure, look at your diet and supplements. If your overall intake of calcium is high, you may need more magnesium. Or vice versa. Always discuss the supplements you want to take with your health provider if you're under a doctor's care for hypertension.

CHAPTER 4

PREVENTING OSTEOPOROSIS

Osteoporosis doesn't just mean having thin bones. It also means that your bones are brittle. Unfortunately, there are no tests for bone brittleness. If you frequently break bones from relatively minor falls, you already know that your bones are brittle. Otherwise, you may have no idea. Doctors tend to rely solely on bone density tests to diagnose osteoporosis because brittleness can't be evaluated. However, your bones may be thinning but they may not be particularly brittle. It depends, to a great degree, on the balance of calcium and magnesium you're getting.

Both calcium and magnesium control the density and brittleness—or flexibility—of bones. Calcium makes bones more brittle, and magnesium makes them more flexible. A good example of this can be seen when you look at the difference between chalk and ivory. Blackboard chalk is calcium carbonate. Drop it and it breaks easily. Ivory is a combination of calcium along with good amounts of magnesium. Drop a piece of ivory and it bounces without breaking. Your bones may be more like chalk, or more like ivory.

An article in *Nutrition Reviews* explains that bones containing less magnesium have larger bone mineral crystals with more perfect shapes. Bones with more magnesium form smaller, more irregular crystals that attach more firmly to one another. The larger, more perfectly shaped crystals are more brittle than the smaller, irregularly shaped bone crystals.

Although your bones contain more calcium than magnesium, magnesium plays an essential role in bone health. It helps transport calcium into the bones and it makes bones stronger. Still, your bones need more than these two minerals. Vitamins C, D, and K, along with boron, manganese, and other trace minerals, are all necessary components of healthy, strong, and dense bone tissue.

Calcium Blood Tests and Your Bones

If a blood tests shows that your calcium is normal, it doesn't mean you have strong bones. Blood tests only test the amount of calcium in your blood, not in your bones. Less than 2 percent of the calcium in your body stays in your blood, so a blood test isn't a good indicator of bone density.

But this small amount of calcium in your blood is so essential for your heart and other functions that if its levels drop, calcium is released from your bones. So a normal calcium blood test could even mean you have less calcium in your bones—especially if your calcium intake is low. Calcium blood tests are used to evaluate parathyroid problems, some kinds of cancers, and bone diseases, but not osteoporosis.

Bone Density Tests and Osteoporosis

There are several types of tests that look at bone density. They can measure the thickness of your bones, but not how fragile or brittle they are. Often, thinner, more porous bones are fragile and break easily. But not always. Bones break when they're brittle, even if they're dense.

Bone density tests vary in their ability to evaluate density. X rays only detect osteoporosis when

25 percent of bone has been lost. Dual X-ray absorptiometry (DEXA) can detect as little as a 3 percent bone loss. Ultrasound tests measure the bone density of your heel, which is a close match to the bone in your spine. (The bone in your heel and spine is different from the bone in your hips.) Therefore, these tests measure the type of bone found in your spine more accurately than the bone found in your hips.

Newer, better tests are constantly being developed. Check with your doctor before having a bone density test and ask what it will and will not show.

High Calcium and Osteoporosis Prevention

Studies don't agree that taking between 1,000 and 1,500 mg of calcium a day protects your bones. In fact, research has shown that large amounts of calcium don't increase bone density. Smaller amounts, it turns out, may be more than enough to prevent bone loss and fractures.

A four-year study published in the *American Journal of Clinical Nutrition* concluded that taking a lot of calcium isn't the answer to the osteoporosis question. Participants took 1,500–2,000 mg of calcium a day. They had a little less bone loss in their arms than women taking less calcium. But the density in their spines and hips didn't improve at all.

A Mayo Clinic osteoporosis study concluded that women who took 1,400 mg of calcium a day had the same amount of bone loss as those who took less than 500 mg a day. What we're seeing now is that current scientific literature suggests that a smaller amount of well-absorbed calcium may be better, along with enough magnesium for optimal calcium absorption.

Susan E. Brown, Ph.D., director of the Osteoporosis Education Project in Syracuse, New York, studied calcium and osteoporosis in women around the world. She discovered that women in underdeveloped countries who had diets with between 200 and 475 mg of calcium a day had strong bones. Women who took 800–1,000 mg a day had more osteoporosis and broken bones.

In spite of the findings that various cultures with low calcium intake have a lower rate of osteoporosis than cultures with high calcium consumption, people still think that high amounts of calcium prevent bone loss. Where did this belief originate? And what was the science behind it? The answer is surprising.

An Explanation of High Calcium Recommendations

Recommendations for taking high amounts of calcium began in 1978 when a poorly conducted, short study conducted by Robert Heaney, M.D., was published *The Journal of Laboratory Clinical Medicine.* In this study, forty-one women in Nebraska kept a one-week food diary and gave Dr. Heaney their dietary history. Their average calcium intake was estimated from this information. Nothing was calculated.

Calcium absorption for these women was also estimated, since there wasn't any way to calculate such general information. The calcium intake for this small group of women averaged around 670 mg a day during this single week. None of the women took as much as 1,500 mg. This study concluded that all women should take more than twice the amount of calcium taken by these Nebraska women. It's not clear how this conclusion was formed.

Marketing Study Results

What happened next shouldn't surprise you. The

dairy industry heard about Dr. Heaney's study and saw an opportunity to sell more high-calcium foods. With the help of the media, they took this one-week study and promoted an increased need for their products to worried women who wanted to protect themselves from osteoporosis. Drug and supplement companies saw that they could use this study to sell more calcium supplements. Today's high calcium recommendations originated from Dr. Heaney's one-week study.

Later, Dr. Heaney published a study on 200 nuns. He observed them for fifteen years and found that the nuns who were on low-calcium diets excreted more calcium each day than they took. Since then, a great many sound scientific studies have concluded just the opposite: when a person's diet is low in calcium, their body conserves and reuses more of it.

In spite of studies concluding that small amounts of calcium can protect the bones when enough magnesium and other nutrients are present, many doctors still recommend the higher amounts. You can now find good studies that say you need a lot of calcium, or just a little. Perhaps both are right and the amount you need depends on your own body's particular needs.

A Look at Individuality

It's easiest to take someone's recommendations and follow them. Especially if they come from an authority like the National Academy of Sciences/ National Research Council or your family doctor. Still, your needs may differ greatly from conclusions found in studies.

Your body theoretically needs 1,000–1,500 mg of calcium and half as much magnesium a day. This is the amount advised by most doctors and found in most supplement formulas. But this high calcium formula may work for only a small number of people. Dr. Abraham discovered that this amount of calcium may actually work against conserving bone as you age. You may need less calcium and more magnesium than you've been told.

Dr. Abraham conducted a small double-blind one-year study and found that women who took 500 mg of calcium and 600 mg of magnesium had an 11 percent increase in bone density. At the end of two years, one woman in the study had an increase in bone density of over 20 percent. This is much higher than any improvement found by taking high amounts of calcium, hormones, or osteoporosis-protective drugs.

Alan R. Gaby, M.D., recommends between 600 and 1,200 mg of calcium for his postmenopausal patients. He uses the higher amount only when he finds specific evidence of a calcium deficiency. Dr. Gaby has found that for the majority of older women who already get about 500 mg of calcium in their diets each day, no supplemental calcium is necessary.

He also recommends taking 250–600 mg of magnesium supplements each day. If your diet is very high in magnesium-rich foods, the lower amount may be enough. If your diet is low in magnesium, you may want to take the higher amount. This higher amount is the quantity that Dr. Abraham's research found to be beneficial. Some foods contain a balance of both minerals. Include them in your diet each day.

Calcium- and Magnesium-rich Foods

Whole grains, beans, nuts, seeds, and green leafy vegetables are all high in both calcium and magnesium.

Calcium Can Contribute to Osteoporosis

Taking too much calcium can create a vicious cycle. Too much calcium keeps you from utilizing magnesium. And you need magnesium to move calcium into your bones. This means that the calcium you're taking is not preserving your bones.

Many people who take high amounts of calcium are under the mistaken impression that it is preventing osteoporosis. In fact, it may be contributing to fragile, porous bones. Without enough magnesium, bone crystals that make up your bone tissues are larger and smoother, resulting in bones that are fragile and weak.

Both magnesium and vitamin D are needed to transport calcium into bone tissues. Neither are found in large enough quantities in high-calcium foods like dairy. They also tend to be low in some supplements. In addition, dairy products contain a lot of phosphorous. Phosphorous is a mineral that blocks calcium from getting into your bones.

The answer is not to take more calcium. It may very well be to take less of a better-absorbed calcium along with more magnesium and vitamin D.

Magnesium Can Protect against Osteoporosis

Magnesium has two roles in bone health. It can make bones more flexible and less brittle. And it can help bone regain some of its lost density. Since osteoporosis is a condition where bones both lose some of their density and become brittle, adding magnesium to your program can protect your bones. Magnesium is often low in women's diets, especially as they age: They tend to eat fewer nuts, seeds, and whole grains in an effort to keep their weight down.

A study on bone density and nutrition, published in the *American Journal of Clinical Nutrition*, found that magnesium was low in the diets and supplements of many postmenopausal women. Their blood levels of magnesium were also low.

This is interesting because blood magnesium levels often don't register as being low even when they are. Therefore, these low blood magnesium levels indicate a significant lack of magnesium.

The researcher on this study also noticed that women with osteoporosis who had spongy bones (that is, bones that lack density and break easily) were low in magnesium. When women took more magnesium, they had fewer broken bones, less bone loss, and an increase in bone density.

Other Bone-Strengthening Nutrients

Vitamin D is called the "sunshine vitamin." This is because your skin uses the ultraviolet rays off the sun to make vitamin D. After calcium and magnesium, this vitamin is the most important nutrient for strong healthy bones. (Vitamin D helps calcium absorption through the intestines.) Vitamin D is often lacking in people who don't spend enough time outdoors. This is particularly true of older people who often spend the majority of their time indoors.

Studies show that when you combine vitamin D with calcium, the rate of hip fracture goes down. One study of nearly 350 women over age seventy were given either 400 IU of vitamin D a day or a placebo for two years. Hipbone density increased 2 to 2.5 percent in the women who took the vitamin. You can get vitamin D by spending time outdoors every day, by taking 400–700 IU of it daily in supplement form, or by getting it from your food. Vitamin D–fortified dairy products, fish, and eggs all contain some of this sunshine vitamin.

International Unit (IU)
An IU, or international unit, is a measure of weight used for fat-soluble vitamins, like vitamins D and E.

Neither calcium nor vitamin D works as well alone as in combination.

Other trace nutrients that help form strong

bones include manganese (15–30 mg per day), boron (3–5 mg per day), zinc (15–20 mg per day), copper (1.5–3 mg per day), folic acid (400–500 mcg per day), vitamin B_6 (50–100 mg per day), vitamin C (500 mg per day), and vitamin K (150–500 mcg per day). Many of these are available in sufficient quantities in a healthy diet. If not, they can be included in a good multivitamin/mineral supplement.

Vitamin K is the vitamin that helps blood clot. Vitamin K is also needed to produce a protein called osteocalcin that helps calcium build bones. Green leafy vegetables are high in vitamin K. But people who are taking Coumadin or other blood thinners must eliminate most vitamin K from their diets and supplements. This lack of vitamin K can contribute to osteoporosis. If you're taking a blood thinner, you'll want to take all the bone-protecting nutrients you safely can.

CHAPTER 5

PMS AND PREGNANCY

Adequate calcium and magnesium are needed to reduce or eliminate premenstrual syndrome (PMS), and are needed during pregnancy. Studies have linked both calcium and magnesium deficiencies to PMS. But compelling evidence from research gynecologist Guy E. Abraham, M.D., and magnesium expert Mildred S. Seelig, M.D., points to a magnesium deficiency in women with emotional premenstrual symptoms like anxiety and depression. And when Dr. Abraham examined the diets of two groups of women with emotional premenstrual symptoms, he found that they ate five times more dairy than other women. It seems that some premenstrual symptoms occur when there is too little magnesium and too much calcium.

With pregnancy comes an increased need for calcium. But pregnant women have an increased ability to absorb it. This means that the amount of calcium in a pregnant woman's diet and supplements does not have to be extremely high because of this increased absorption. Pregnant women also have a need for enough magnesium to prevent them from going

PMS
Premenstrual syndrome (PMS) consists of a number of physical or emotional symptoms that occur during the week before menstruation. They usually disappear with menstruation or after it begins.

into early labor. They also need enough calcium and magnesium to prevent a condition called preeclampsia.

Preeclampsia
A complication of pregnancy that can include high blood pressure, water retention, and protein in the urine.

A woman's need for various nutrients changes during different life cycles. Menstruation and pregnancy are two cycles when it is particularly important to get sufficient calcium and magnesium.

Causes of PMS

Hormone levels fluctuate before, during, and after the menstrual cycle. This causes an ever-changing need for a number of nutrients—particularly calcium and magnesium.

It appears that hormonal and nutrient excesses and deficiencies lead to premenstrual symptoms. Some are physical—like tender breasts and weight gain. Others are emotional. Each has their causes that often stem from nutrient deficiencies. Dr. Abraham has separated PMS into four categories: anxiety, depression, cravings, and hydration (water retention). The first two categories are emotional; the second two are primarily physical.

Emotional premenstrual symptoms like anxiety, depression, and mood swings are often a sign of a magnesium deficiency, calcium excess, or both. A study published in the *Journal of Orthomolecular Psychiatry* found a connection between high-dairy diets and aggressiveness in girls. High amounts of calcium interfere with the body's ability to break down sugar. Large quantities of sugar in the bloodstream, which causes magnesium excretion, can contribute to mood changes and aggressiveness. This may be one explanation for how a high-dairy diet negatively affects emotional premenstrual symptoms.

Magnesium's Role in PMS

Estrogen and progesterone are the primary hormones that regulate menstruation. Their production increases and decreases around the monthly menstrual cycle. Hormones can greatly influence your moods. In fact, estrogen contributes to premenstrual symptoms of anxiety and depression. It also increases magnesium excretion just when it is needed the most. Magnesium plays an important role in these monthly hormonal changes.

Production of estrogen and progesterone increases during a normal menstrual cycle. But to make progesterone, a hormone that has sedative effects, the body needs enough magnesium.

Low levels of progesterone appear to be responsible for premenstrual symptoms like anxiety and depression. In some women, progesterone levels remain low because there are not enough nutrients, like magnesium, present to increase them. High-magnesium foods, like whole grains and beans, contain good amounts of vitamin B_6. This vitamin helps the body make more progesterone.

Magnesium also plays an important role in the production of brain chemicals. Before menstruation, the body makes a number of stimulating chemicals called neurotransmitters that can lead to anxiety. Magnesium helps the brain make a calming neurotransmitter, dopamine, which counteracts the effects of the stimulating neurotransmitters.

Neurotransmitter
One of a number of chemicals used by the nervous system and in the brain to send messages. Their balance affects your mood.

All stress, like the hormonal fluctuations caused by the menstrual cycle, results in your body excreting magnesium faster than normal. This is another reason why women need extra magnesium before menstruation. One possible signal of a magnesium deficiency is craving chocolate. The common phenomenon of chocolate craving before menstruation may be your body's way of telling you it needs more magnesium.

Chocolate Craving and Magnesium Deficiency

There are a number of reasons why people crave chocolate, including a magnesium deficiency. The reason is simple: Chocolate contains some of the highest amounts of magnesium of any food.

But eating a lot of chocolate to raise your magnesium levels is not the answer. Foods containing chocolate are high in sugar and fat, as well as in magnesium. The sugar causes drowsiness, difficulty concentrating, nervousness, and water retention—other premenstrual symptoms. The fat binds with magnesium making it difficult to absorb. However, a chocolate craving may help you recognize that at some stressful times, your body needs more magnesium.

When Calcium Helps PMS

Some women with PMS may need more calcium, rather than more magnesium. One study had women take either 1,200 mg of calcium a day or a placebo. After three months, almost half of the women who took the calcium supplement had fewer PMS symptoms.

Placebo
An inactive substance that is used as a control in clinical studies instead of a drug or nutrient.

The same researchers had conducted a smaller study with similar results. In both studies, they used calcium carbonate, a poorly absorbed form of calcium. It is possible that smaller amounts of a better-absorbed calcium, like calcium citrate, would give similar results without risking a calcium overload that could lead to arthritis and heart disease.

Most researchers have found that increasing

magnesium is more effective than increasing calcium for women with PMS. This is especially true for those who eat a lot of dairy products—foods that are high in calcium and low in magnesium.

Mildred S. Seelig, M.D., points out that since calcium impairs the absorption of magnesium, any time you take extra calcium you also need to take more magnesium. Today's emphasis on calcium has encouraged many women to eat diets that create a wider and wider gap between calcium and magnesium balance, creating a greater and greater magnesium deficiency.

Calcium Needs during Pregnancy and Nursing

Calcium requirements for women increase during pregnancy and lactation, but that's not the whole story. In fact, concentrating on calcium can be misleading. At times when more calcium is needed, like during pregnancy, the body is able to absorb more from both foods and supplements.

Nature knows that fetuses need calcium to form bones, and that mother's milk needs to provide babies with plenty of calcium for the same reason. Doctors know this, too. This is why the revised U.S.-Canadian dietary guidelines no longer recommend that pregnant or lactating women take extra calcium. The recommendation is for 1,000 mg of calcium a day. This includes all calcium in foods and supplements, not just supplements.

Calcium and magnesium are both helpful in preventing leg cramps associated with pregnancy. Once again, the idea is to get enough, but not too much, of each mineral. And in looking at calcium requirements during pregnancy, it's easy to overlook the importance of magnesium. (See the discussion "How Magnesium and Calcium Help Preeclampsia" on page 49.)

Magnesium and Pregnancy

Long-term studies indicate that at least 450 mg of magnesium a day is needed to keep both mothers and their fetuses healthy. Once again, some women may need much more. Dr. Seelig reports that a woman who had a number of uncomplicated pregnancies and gave birth to healthy babies needed to take as much as 600 mg of magnesium a day during the last half of her pregnancy. When she took less than 300 mg a day, her doctor found her to be deficient in magnesium.

Magnesium is a valuable nutrient for pregnant women because it can prevent premature birth and reduce pregnancy-related constipation. In a four-month study of more than 550 pregnant women, those who took magnesium supplements had fewer premature babies. In addition, fewer mothers were hospitalized before giving birth, and fewer newborn babies needed to be in intensive care. Naturopath Tori Hudson, N.D., Professor at the National College of Naturopathic Medicine in Portland, Oregon, explains that the best time for pregnant women to increase their magnesium is during their first trimester if they want to prevent low-birth weight in their babies.

Many women now take extra magnesium to prevent constipation during pregnancy. Gynecologist Uzzi Reiss, M.D., has told some of his patients they could take magnesium to bowel tolerance during their pregnancies to avoid this pressure-related constipation. Some of his patients took as much as 1,000 mg of supplementary magnesium a day in addition to whatever amounts they got from their diets. Before increasing magnesium, pregnant women should always check with their doctors.

A number of studies have shown that a magnesium deficiency is common in both normal pregnancies and those complicated by diabetes or high blood pressure. And, as mentioned previously, sufficient magnesium can help prevent preeclampsia.

How Magnesium and Calcium Help Preeclampsia

Preeclampsia can occur during the last trimester of pregnancy when blood pressure is elevated. Among other symptoms, it may result in kidney damage and water retention. Preeclampsia can also restrict blood flow to the fetus. This limits the amount of oxygen and nourishment available to the developing baby.

Magnesium may counteract the constriction of blood vessels. These blood vessels need calcium to contract, but they also need sufficient magnesium to relax and open up. Magnesium acts as a calcium-channel blocker to help regulate blood pressure. Without high blood pressure, preeclampsia is rare.

In addition to bed rest, a high-protein diet, and at times taking medications to reduce high blood pressure, magnesium is the major treatment of choice for this complication of pregnancy. However, too little calcium can also lead to preeclampsia. So once again, the proper balance of these two minerals is of vital importance.

How Much Calcium and Magnesium Is Needed during Pregnancy?

The amount of calcium and magnesium needed by a pregnant woman depends, in part, on the absorbability of the calcium in the diet and the supplement. When you take a well-absorbed form of calcium like calcium citrate or calcium malate, you need less than when you're taking calcium carbonate or dolomite. Pregnant women who consume 500–750 mg of good quality calcium each day in their diets and supplements should have plenty for themselves and their babies. This can be achieved either with or without dairy products.

Dr. Seelig recommends that pregnant women take 450 mg of magnesium. This is slightly higher than the 350 mg suggested by the current RDAs, and less than the 1,000 mg some physicians give their patients to counteract constipation.

It makes sense to take some extra magnesium, since this is a mineral that is excreted when we're under stress, and pregnancy is physiologically, as well as emotionally, stressful. There may be fewer times in a woman's life when her body is under more stress than during pregnancy.

CHAPTER 6

COUNTERACTING DEPRESSION AND FATIGUE

It takes a complex series of biochemical activities to convert food into energy. And another series of actions to produce brain chemicals that give you a feeling of either well-being or depression. In both cases, you need enough specific nutrients to turn your food either into energy or into mood-elevating brain chemicals. These specific nutrients include calcium and magnesium.

One of the most important nutrients to help you feel energetic and happy is magnesium. But once again, while magnesium has been recognized as being of primary importance, some studies indicate that calcium needs must be met, as well. Although you may need to emphasize magnesium over calcium to counteract depression and fatigue, these two minerals work so closely together that you can't consider one without the other.

Depression

A common mood disorder that may include poor appetite, insomnia or excessive sleeping, lack of interest, fatigue, feelings of worthlessness, and an inability to concentrate.

How Calcium Affects Depression

While calcium is not commonly known to affect moods, two preliminary studies, published in the *Journal of Orthomolecular Psychiatry*, indicate it may help reduce depression. These studies took a group of college students, both male and female, and gave them either 1,000 mg of calcium with 600 IU of vitamin D twice a day for a month, or a placebo. The students who took the calcium and vitamin D had half as much depression as those who took the placebo.

On the other hand, too much calcium can cause depression in some people. A number of studies have associated personality changes and depression in psychiatric patients with high calcium levels. Too much calcium can contribute to depression, irritability, and a lack of initiative.

More studies on the connection between calcium and depression are needed, but calcium may play a role in your mood. Too little, or too much, can affect the way you feel. If you suffer from depression, you may want to have your calcium levels evaluated by your doctor both through blood tests and by looking at your dietary calcium intake. Take a look at how much calcium you get each day and see how your mood changes if you take less or more. Calcium's role in depression is unclear at this time. Magnesium's role is better understood.

How Magnesium Helps Reduce Depression

Magnesium, along with vitamin B_6, helps produce serotonin, an important brain neurotransmitter. Serotonin is considered to be a natural antidepressant, and a serotonin deficiency is one common cause for depression. In these cases, when a lack of serotonin contributes to depression, taking more magnesium can be helpful.

Psychiatrist Hyla Cass, M.D., explains that low serotonin production can cause a number of symptoms from depression to obsessive thinking, anxiety, violent behavior, PMS, and alcohol or drug abuse.

Many medical doctors treat a serotonin-deficiency depression with a class of drugs called SSRIs (selective serotonin reuptake inhibitors). These drugs, which include Prozac, Zoloft, and Paxil, make serotonin more available to brain cells. But certain amino acids like l-tryptophan or its derivative 5-HTP can have the same effect. However, these amino acids need to be taken along with magnesium for them to work.

Amino Acids
A group of organic compounds that are the building blocks of protein. Along with vitamins, minerals, and enzymes, they help make other needed chemicals, like neurotransmitters.

Since serotonin can't get from the bloodstream into the brain, your brain needs to constantly make this chemical. The raw ingredients needed to make a substance like serotonin are called precursors. Magnesium is a precursor to serotonin production.

Tryptophan, 5-HTP, Magnesium, and Depression

To counteract many forms of depression, you may need more serotonin. But before serotonin can be produced, your body needs to have enough tryptophan and magnesium. Here's how serotonin production works.

Tryptophan is an amino acid that gets into your brain where it is converted into serotonin. But first it needs to be changed into a chemical called 5-HTP (5-hydroxytryptophan). Then, 5-HTP needs helpers—mainly magnesium and vitamin B_6.

These three nutrients—5-HTP, magnesium, and vitamin B_6—work together to help make serotonin, a neurotransmitter that carries messages throughout your brain, which affects your mood, sleep, and other body functions.

An article in *Alternative Medicine Review* examined a Swiss study of more than 500 participants with a variety of types of depression. Some of the participants were seriously depressed while others were just a little sad. Everyone was given 5-HTP, and the study concluded that this nutrient worked even better than SSRI drugs in reducing depression.

You may not need to take 5-HTP. Since your body needs magnesium to make serotonin, you might just want to begin by taking more magnesium. If that's not enough, you can always try adding 5-HTP. Psychiatrist Priscilla Slagle, M.D., who has worked extensively with natural solutions to depression, notes that people who are depressed may need to take as much as 100–500 mg of magnesium orotate three times a day. Other forms of magnesium should work as well as the orotate.

If you decide next to take 5-HTP, which is better absorbed and easier to find than tryptophan, Dr. Slagle has found that healthy people need 100–200 mg of 5-HTP (or 1,000–2,000 mg of tryptophan) a day. Someone who is depressed, she says, may need even more. She gives her patients an average of 300–400 mg of 5-HTP a day. But don't just run out and buy this supplement. Talk with your doctor first. It could be just what you need, or just the reverse. If you sleep a lot when you're depressed, for instance, you may not need tryptophan or 5-HTP at all.

Amino acids are powerful nutrients, and the balance between all of them is important. You don't want too much of one and not enough of another. Magnesium is a bit different. It's clear that so many people are magnesium deficient; therefore, adding more magnesium to your diet and taking supplements is likely to do one of the following: help, have no effect, or cause loose stools. So, it's a pretty safe nutrient to try for depression.

Fighting Fatigue

Magnesium is also an important ingredient in creating energy. Without enough magnesium, you can feel tired and drained. You need enough magnesium for your body to turn all of the sugars in your diet into energy. This includes cookies, fruit, honey, and all starches (carbohydrates) that eventually turn into sugar.

You also need magnesium to give your muscles their strength. If you have weak muscles, it may be because you're not exercising enough. Or it could be due to a deficiency of either magnesium or its partner in energy production: potassium. Or you could need both.

Use Potassium Along with Magnesium

Fatigue and muscle weakness are the most common symptoms of a chronic potassium deficiency. But potassium doesn't work alone. It needs magnesium. In fact, a magnesium deficiency may be one reason why you need more potassium. If your potassium and magnesium levels are both low, taking more potassium without also boosting your magnesium intake is often not enough. Taking potassium by itself could cause more magnesium to be excreted in your urine. If it seems like you may need more potassium, make sure you're getting enough magnesium, as well.

Dr Alan R. Gaby found that when fatigue is due to low potassium, taking a potassium/magnesium aspartate supplement often helps. Aspartic acid is an excellent chemical to transport both potassium and magnesium into cells. Dr. Gaby noticed that between 75 and 91 percent of participants in several double-blind studies who took this combined supplement had much more energy after taking it. Talk with your doctor about the advisability of using potassium/magnesium aspartate supplements for low energy. The amount suggested is 70 mg of magnesium aspartate and 99 mg of potassium aspartate three times a day.

Potassium can be found in a healthy diet. It is abundant in all vegetables, but especially dark green leafy ones. Orange juice, whole grains, sunflower seeds, and potatoes are also high in this mineral. But alcohol, caffeine, and sodium all increase the excretion of potassium.

Chronic Fatigue and Magnesium

Chronic fatigue is more than a feeling of lethargy. It is a complex syndrome that often includes muscle and/or joint pain, headaches, poor sleep, poor memory, and a sore throat. Rest doesn't help people with chronic fatigue feel better. Medical doctors are often puzzled by how to treat their chronic fatigue patients unless they are well versed in nutrition. Then, they find magnesium can frequently help.

Scientific studies on magnesium's effect on chronic fatigue have resulted in mixed results. Some say magnesium helps; others say it doesn't. When it does work, it is impressive in alleviating some of the debilitating fatigue that prevents people with this condition from accomplishing even the simplest of daily tasks.

It appears that chronic fatigue patients who have low magnesium levels respond positively to taking additional amounts of this mineral. And these are the majority of chronic fatigue patients. A lack of magnesium has been associated with fatigue, pain, weakness, muscle spasms, irritability, and numbness—all symptoms of chronic fatigue. The only people who should avoid taking extra magnesium are people with chronic kidney failure. Very few of them have chronic fatigue.

Jacob Teitelbaum, M.D., a leading researcher in the field of chronic fatigue, suggests that people who have either fatigue or chronic fatigue syndrome should take magnesium supplements. It will either do nothing or result in more energy and a reduction in other chronic fatigue symptoms within two or three weeks. But magnesium supplements are not the only answer. Dr. Teitelbaum stresses that a healthy diet, along with magnesium, is essential.

CHAPTER 7

OTHER USES FOR CALCIUM AND MAGNESIUM

The amount of calcium and magnesium you get affects a wide variety of health conditions. This balance of calcium to magnesium affects stress, twitching muscles, hyperactivity, muscle pain including fibromyalgia, and headaches. While you need enough calcium to keep your bones healthy and your body functioning properly, taking additional magnesium is often even more helpful in a number of conditions that affect the muscles. This is because magnesium helps muscles to relax.

Also, magnesium has been found to be low in many people with diabetes. So anyone who has diabetes should have their magnesium intakes evaluated, and consider increasing this mineral in their diets. People with a family history of colon cancer, on the other hand, may benefit from taking extra calcium. Once again, your body's particular needs, rather than a "one size fits all" approach, help determine how much of each of these minerals you should be getting. Look at your diet and your health to see whether you need more calcium, magnesium, or both.

How Magnesium Helps Stress

Whenever you're under stress, your body excretes more magnesium than usual. This is a normal stress response. When you're under any kind of stress, your body produces particular hormones to help you handle it. These hormones contribute to a magnesium deficiency by increasing magnesium excretion.

Your brain needs plenty of energy when you're under stress to help you cope and make wise decisions, and glucose is the brain's energy source. But to turn foods into glucose, you need enough magnesium. Your nervous system also needs extra magnesium when you're under stress. You need plenty of magnesium every day, but especially whenever you're stressed and nervous. Foods high in magnesium include whole grains, beans, nuts, seeds, and green vegetables. One reason why it's important to eat very well when you're under stress is that a healthy diet is high in magnesium.

Stress
Anything that disturbs your balance. Stress can be emotional, mental, physical, thermal (too hot or too cold), or economic.

Mildred S. Seelig, M.D., explains that stress causes fatty acids to be released. These fats attach themselves to magnesium. When magnesium gets stuck to fatty acids, it isn't well absorbed.

Other nutrients besides magnesium are needed when you're under stress. They include B vitamins, zinc, and vitamin C. These vitamins and minerals can also be found in a high-magnesium diet.

Restless Legs

If your legs twitch and you can't stop them from twitching, you may have a condition called restless leg syndrome (RLS). This neurological condition can include tingling, itching, burning, and other uncomfortable sensations that are often relieved by walking. While some people have restless legs during the day, their symptoms are often worse at night. This makes it difficult to get a good night's sleep.

The cause of RLS isn't understood, but we know it involves a problem in the nervous system, a system dependent on getting enough magnesium. Both calcium and magnesium are needed to strengthen your muscle function. And both are needed by your central nervous system. But additional magnesium is often needed even more than calcium.

A number of anecdotal reports indicate that magnesium supplementation reduces RLS. This makes sense, since a deficiency of magnesium can increase muscle excitability, or twitching. If you have restless leg syndrome, you can begin by boosting your dietary and supplemental magnesium. Loose stools are a sign that you're taking more magnesium than your body can handle. If this occurs, reduce your intake to an amount that causes comfortably loose stools. If your symptoms don't improve, see if additional calcium improves or worsens your condition.

A study published in the journal *Sleep* reported a 75 to 85 percent improvement in sleeping with RLS patients who took magnesium. Previously, twitching legs awakened them or prevented them from getting to sleep. Magnesium was most helpful in people with mild to moderate restless leg syndrome.

A deficiency of folic acid has also been associated with RLS. Taking 400 mcg twice a day with a little vitamin B_{12} often helps reduce twitching. So does eliminating coffee and other sources of caffeine.

Restless Children

Hyperactivity can affect children, adolescents, and adults. It is now popularly called ADHD, or attention-deficit hyperactivity disorder. While hyperactivity may be caused by prenatal alcohol or drug abuse, a reaction to certain foods or medications, or lead poisoning, it can also be due to a need for specific nutrients. Calcium and magnesium are two of the most important nutrients to counteract hyperactivity.

Acupuncturist Janet Zand, LAc, OMD, suggests that children aged five to seven who have ADHD begin by taking one teaspoonful of a liquid calcium and magnesium supplement once a day. For children aged seven to ten, she suggests this amount twice a day. Children over ten, she says, should take one tablespoon once or twice a day. After two months, Dr. Zand reduces this supplement to five times a week for three more months. Then the supplement is stopped. Hyperactive children have an increased need for calcium since their bones are forming. Adults may find a reduction in restlessness by taking magnesium alone. Magnesium without additional calcium may work for children, also, if their diets contain dairy and other sources of calcium.

In a six-month study published in *Magnesium Research Journal,* half the children with ADHD were given 200 mg of magnesium a day. The control group took nothing. The children who took magnesium had a noticeably greater reduction in their hyperactivity. There was no change in the control group.

Other nutrients besides magnesium appear to be helpful in counteracting ADHD. Hyperactive children often need a vitamin B complex to help support their nervous systems. But magnesium may be a significant part of the puzzle.

Headaches

Headaches can be triggered by a number of factors including food sensitivities, low blood sugar, and stress. But migraine headaches, including premenstrual migraines, may be caused by low magnesium.

In a study published in *Contemporary Nutrition,* 3,000 female migraine sufferers were given 100–200 mg of magnesium a day. Eighty percent of the participants had a reduction in the frequency and severity of their migraines.

Another study, published in a headache journal, *Cephalagia,* observed eighty people for one month. Then, half were given 600 mg of magnesium a day for three months while the other half were given a placebo. Within nine weeks, magnesium reduced the severity and length of migraines in more than 40 percent of the participants. While it's true that magnesium didn't provide an immediate solution, it was a considerable help to a good percentage of migraine sufferers. And it allowed them to reduce their migraine medicine, as well.

Some migraines are associated with menstruation. Dr. Abraham and his colleagues conducted a study on premenstrual syndrome (PMS) with more than two dozen women. They measured both serum magnesium and red blood cell magnesium in all participants. Women with premenstrual migraines had low red blood cell magnesium levels although their serum magnesium levels were normal. Serum magnesium is the most common way of measuring magnesium. It is not as accurate as red blood cell magnesium—a test that is rarely done because of the expense.

Tight muscles may contribute to everyday tension headaches. Because magnesium relaxes all muscles, it may be helpful for this common variety of headaches. If you have frequent tension headaches, you may want to increase your magnesium.

Fibromyalgia

No one knows what causes fibromyalgia. But this painful condition results in fatigue, along with stiffness and aching in muscles and soft tissues—areas that contain high concentrations of magnesium. In fact, there's an overlapping between fibromyalgia and chronic fatigue syndrome. In fibromyalgia, there's more pain; in chronic fatigue there's more fatigue.

Jorge D. Flechas, M.D., a physician from North Carolina, measured red blood cell magnesium in fibromyalgia patients. The results were stunning. He found low magnesium in twelve out of thirteen patients.

One theory about the relationship between magnesium and fibromyalgia is that the painful muscles may not have enough magnesium to relax them. Another concerns a connection between pain and serotonin. We know that fibromyalgia patients have low levels of serotonin. And when serotonin is chronically low, pain feels even more severe. Without enough magnesium, your brain can't make serotonin.

Magnesium is an important nutrient in the production of a compound called adenosine triphosphate (ATP). ATP furnishes energy to muscles. Both magnesium and malic acid, a substance found in apples and some other fruits, are needed to make ATP. It is very possible that fibromyalgia is a result of a deficiency of both magnesium and malic acid.

Dr. Flechas conducted several studies treating fibromyalgia patients with a combination of magnesium and malic acid. The patients who took 300–600 mg of magnesium, and 1,200–2,400 mg of malic acid, each day had less pain within one or two months. Other controlled studies showed a 50 percent reduction in fibromyalgia pain in two months using both supplements. Two days after the subjects stopped taking magnesium with malic acid, their pain returned. While not all studies show this degree of effectiveness, it is safe enough and inexpensive enough to try for several months to see if it works for you.

Magnesium and Diabetes

Magnesium is the most common mineral deficiency in insulin-dependent diabetes. In fact, low magnesium is more common in people with both insulin-dependent (type 1) and non-insulin-dependent (type 2) diabetes than in any other group of people. The reason is simple.

A balance is needed between insulin and magnesium to regulate blood sugar. Your body needs magnesium to secrete enough insulin to keep your blood sugar level, and insulin helps transport magnesium into your cells. In a seven-year study of 14,000 middle-aged people called the Atherosclerosis Risk in Communities Study (ARIC), people who had the lowest magnesium levels were twice as likely to get diabetes as those with the highest magnesium levels. To prevent or support the treatment of diabetes, getting enough magnesium is key.

Magnesium and Type-2 Diabetes

Type-2 diabetes, or non-insulin dependent diabetes, is often a result of obesity in later years. Type-2 diabetes often can be controlled by diet and weight loss. But additional magnesium helps.

Maria De Lourdes Lima, M.D., and her associates conducted a study in Brazil with more than 124 people with type-2 diabetes. Twenty-five to 38 percent of the participants had low magnesium. Some diabetics in this study were given additional magnesium, while others were given a placebo. The magnesium was given to participants whether or not they had low magnesium levels. Magnesium helped improve blood sugar regulation, especially in people with neuropathy (damage to nerve tissue) or with heart disease.

Dr. Lima and her colleagues noticed that the participants in this study had to be given higher than usual doses of magnesium to get results. In fact, they needed 800–1,600 mg a day. If you have type-2 diabetes, you may want to talk with your doctor about adding more magnesium to your diet and supplement program.

Diabetic Neuropathy
A condition that occurs in some people who have diabetes that can cause muscle pain, tingling, and numbness, commonly found in the legs. It can also occur in the hands and arms.

The amount you need may be quite a bit lower than this. Naturopath Kathi Head, N.D., suggests 200–500 mg of supplemental magnesium a day.

Calcium's Role in Diabetes

Too much calcium is more likely to be a problem for people with diabetes than too little calcium. Several studies indicate that diabetes may accelerate the deposit of calcium in the walls of arteries. This can lead to high blood pressure and heart disease—conditions that are common in people with diabetes. Don't overdo dietary calcium by eating a lot of dairy products. Even low-fat and nonfat dairy contains high amounts of calcium. Keep your calcium supplements low, around 500 mg a day, and be sure to take enough magnesium with it.

As you've learned, magnesium is a natural calcium-channel blocker. It prevents calcium from adhering to artery walls. For this reason, it appears to be even more important for people with diabetes to concentrate on getting enough magnesium. And keep calcium intake reasonable, not high, to guard against an excess of calcium, and to prevent these calcium deposits.

Colon Cancer

Extra calcium may be important if you have a family history of colon cancer. The connection between this mineral and colon cancer is just now starting to be understood.

Both dietary fats and bile, a substance produced in the liver to help digest them, can irritate the intestines. This, in turn, causes a buildup of protective cells, like a Band-Aid. But this buildup of cells is abnormal, and in a small but significant number of people, it could lead to cancer.

A study published in *The New England Journal of Medicine* found that calcium supplements slowed down cell growth in the intestines most successfully in people with a family history of colon cancer. There seems to be a genetic tendency for this buildup in some families. When this particular subgroup of people increased their calcium from 700 mg to 1,250 mg a day, fewer "Band-Aid" cells were made. Both cancerous and precancerous cells grew faster in people with a genetic tendency for colon cancer who ate a high-fat, low-calcium diet.

A more recent study by the Calcium Polyp Prevention Study Group, also published in *The New England Journal of Medicine,* found that taking calcium supplements could be helpful to people who have had colon cancer in the past. This study took more than 900 people with a recent history of colon cancer and gave half of them 1,200 mg of calcium a day and the other half a placebo. At the end of this four-year study, those people who had taken extra calcium had fewer recurrences of colon cancer than those on the placebo. In this particular study, dietary fat and dietary calcium had no effect; only calcium supplements had an effect.

If you have a concern about colon cancer, reduce the amount of all fats in your diet. If you have a family history of this disease, or have had colon cancer yourself, consider increasing your supplemental calcium.

CHAPTER 8

HOW TO GET
ENOUGH CALCIUM

Calcium absorption is even more important than the amount of calcium you get. You may think that if a food contains 100 mg of calcium, then 100 mg of calcium is absorbed and available to your bones and other tissues. But this isn't true. Only a fraction of the calcium in different foods is useable. It's the same with calcium supplements. Some are well absorbed; others are not. Whatever your body can't use becomes a potential problem.

When calcium isn't absorbed into your bones and other tissues, it can contribute to heart disease, kidney stones, and arthritis. Taking high amounts of calcium to prevent bone loss does not guarantee strong bones. The key is to take enough, but not too much, calcium. And it's just as important to get enough magnesium and other cofactors to help your body use the calcium in your supplements and diet.

Many nondairy sources of dietary calcium contain these cofactors. Dairy does not. Look for foods, such as whole grains, dark green vegetables, and beans, that have both calcium and magnesium for best absorption.

To evaluate your daily intake, count all the calcium in your foods and supplements. Not just the amount in the pills you take. And be sure to include enough magnesium whenever you take calcium. This means doing more than merely taking a handful of calcium supplements or eating a lot of dairy.

Assessing Your Calcium Needs

Not everyone needs 1,000–1,500 mg of supplemental calcium a day. The total amount of calcium your body needs comes from both diet and supplements. Still many people eat dairy and other high-calcium foods while taking 1,000 mg or more of a calcium supplement. As you've learned, this can be dangerous.

To decide how much calcium you may need, first look at your personal and family health histories. Some disorders are a sign of low or poorly absorbed calcium. These include arthritis, heart disease, and osteoporosis. If you have any of these health problems, look to see whether you need to take more calcium than you've been taking, or a better-absorbed form.

Next, look for reasons why calcium may not be well absorbed. These include not getting magnesium and having low amounts of hydrochloric acid (stomach acid). Acid is needed to break down and use both calcium and magnesium. For this reason, calcium in antacids is not as well absorbed as other forms. See the discussion "Antacids and Calcium Absorption" on page 14.

There is compelling evidence to suggest that high amounts of calcium are not necessary and may even contribute to health problems. If you're taking a well-absorbed form, you may need much less than the amount most people recommend.

Look for signs of calcium excess. If you're taking too much calcium, you may have muscle cramps, fibromyalgia, irregular heartbeat (arrhythmias), restless leg syndrome, or premenstrual syndrome (PMS). In these cases, symptoms may improve by lowering supplemental calcium to 500 mg a day.

If you are determining how much calcium your child needs, remember that children and adolescents, whose bones are still forming and growing, need more calcium than adults do.

Dairy Products as a Source of Calcium

We've been taught that dairy products are a good source of dietary calcium. In fact, we've heard so much about dairy that few people realize that there are other calcium-rich foods. But dairy has limitations that you should consider when you're evaluating your calcium intake.

Dairy is rich in calcium, with very little magnesium, which is needed to help move calcium into your bones. So, a diet containing dairy should also include high-magnesium foods like nuts, seeds, whole grains, beans, and green vegetables.

Dairy is also high in phosphorous, and while you need phosphorous for strong bones, too much can interfere with calcium absorption and cause increased calcium excretion. The typical American diet contains too much phosphorous. High-phosphorous foods include animal protein and colas. You need equal amounts of calcium and phosphorous for healthy bones. While small amounts of dairy may have its place in a diet designed to help bones stay strong, high-dairy diets may not be protecting your bones as much as you think—especially if you're eating a lot of protein and drinking colas.

Limitations of Dairy

The association between eating a lot of dairy and osteoporosis is not what you think. People who live in countries with the highest dairy consumption—the United States, Great Britain, and Sweden—have the highest amount of osteoporosis. People on diets low in dairy, like Asians and many Africans, have stronger bones. Clearly, dairy is not the solution for strong bones.

In addition, not everyone can digest dairy. Lactose intolerance is another reason why dairy is not the only, or best, source of dietary calcium for many people. Yogurt is one form of dairy that is low in lactose and easier for people with lactose intolerance to digest.

Lactose Intolerance
The inability to digest milk sugar. This intolerance leads to bloating and cramping after eating milk, cheese, and other dairy products.

Drinking milk is not natural. Michael Klaper, M.D., points out that of all the animals on earth, humans are the only species that drink the milk of other species. We're also the only species to drink milk after we're weaned. It appears that nature is trying to tell us something, but we're not listening. The voice of vested interest groups, like the American Dairy Association, are shouting in our ears, preventing us from listening to other, more logical, messages.

Scientific Studies and Dairy

There have been numerous studies that looked at dairy products and osteoporosis. One impressive twelve-year study of 78,000 women, published in the *American Journal of Public Health,* had a surprising finding. Women who drank two or more glasses of milk a day had more hip fractures than those who drank it once a week or less.

Cardiologist Kurt Oster, M.D., has published studies that found that an enzyme in cow's milk could lead to heart disease. This enzyme damages cell membranes in the arteries. Normally, digestive juices destroy this enzyme. But when the milk is homogenized, the enzyme can get into your arteries and cause considerable damage. Since most dairy products are homogenized, it might be wise to limit dairy products to protect against heart disease.

In an article published in the *International Journal of Cardiology*, Stephen Seely, M.D., points out that our need for calcium decreases as we age. He found that a diet high in calcium could lead to small amounts of the mineral getting into soft tissues, like the aorta, resulting in heart disease. He also found that high blood pressure does not exist in countries where calcium intake is low. (See "Calcium's Role in a Healthy Heart" on page 31.)

Dietary Sources of Calcium

Calcium is everywhere, and all calcium counts toward your daily dose. Beans, whole grains, green vegetables, and fish (with small edible bones, like canned salmon) all contain good amounts of calcium. Canned salmon, for instance, has 350–550 mg of calcium. Fresh salmon, without bones, has none since the calcium in fish comes from the bones.

Many common foods have good amounts of this important mineral. A cup of broccoli has 178 mg, and a cup of most any kind of beans supplies at least 130 mg. Some contain much more. Half a cup of garbanzo beans, for instance, will give you more than 200 mg of calcium. Half a cup of tofu (soybean curd) contains 100–300 mg. Even an orange has 56 mg. Of all nuts, almonds are highest in calcium content. One tablespoon of almond butter has 40 mg, while an ounce of the nuts themselves contains nearly 80 mg.

Many foods have smaller amounts of calcium. Add them up at the end of the day and you will find your calcium intake is much higher than you thought. For instance, a cup of blackberries (46 mg), a kiwi fruit (74 mg), or a single dried fig (19 mg) added to a salad, broccoli, and a few nuts gives you a good amount of useable calcium.

Absorbing Dietary Calcium

Contrary to popular belief, calcium from plant products is well absorbed. Registered dietician Vesanto Melina points out that 50 to 70 percent of the calcium found in cooked vegetables like broccoli and kale gets into tissues. Only 32 percent of calcium from dairy products, on the other hand, is used.

You can increase the absorption of calcium by soaking beans overnight, sprouting seeds (like sunflower seeds), roasting nuts, and cooking grains. And you can get more useable calcium just by chewing better.

As mentioned previously, when you chew your food well, your body secretes hydrochloric acid (HCl), the acid made in your stomach that helps you use calcium, magnesium, iron, and protein. As you've learned, it's not a good idea to take antacids when you eat calcium-rich foods or when you're taking calcium supplements. Antacids neutralize stomach acid and lowers calcium absorption. Add acidic foods like lemon juice, orange juice, vinegar, or tomatoes to high-calcium foods, or when you take calcium supplements.

Limit your calcium intake to about 500 mg at any one time. This is the amount found in many healthy meals. Your body will use more calcium if you take it frequently in small quantities rather than if you take large amounts all at once. Finally, choose a calcium supplement that is easy for your body to use.

Evaluating Calcium Supplements

Some calcium supplements may contain lead, a harmful heavy metal. Lead has been found in bone meal and dolomite. Avoid these forms. Lead is lowest in supplements where calcium is attached to citrate, fumarate, succinate, or aspartate, or amino acid chelate. In addition to not containing lead, they are better absorbed than calcium carbonate, an inexpensive and frequently used calcium source.

To give you an idea of the absorbability of calcium supplements, look at calcium carbonate versus calcium citrate. About 45 percent of calcium in a citrate form can be absorbed by people with low stomach acid. Only 4 percent of calcium carbonate is available to these same people. Once again, because acid is needed to utilize calcium, antacids are not a good source of calcium.

Calcium hydroxyapatite is a popular ingredient in several bone-building formulas. But naturopath Tori Hudson, N.D., points out that this form of calcium is simply purified bone meal and may also contain lead. While claims of superior absorption have been made for calcium hydroxyapatite, Dr. Hudson finds it is even less absorbable than calcium carbonate.

The best forms of calcium supplements are calcium citrate, calcium malate, calcium fumarate, calcium succinate, calcium aspartate, and calcium amino acid chelate.

CHAPTER 9

HOW TO GET ENOUGH MAGNESIUM

You may not be getting enough magnesium in your diet, especially if you have signs of a magnesium deficiency. As you may recall, high-magnesium foods include nuts, seeds, whole grains, beans, and dark green vegetables. Even if you eat these foods every day, you may be losing valuable magnesium due to stress, a high-fat diet, colas, or too much vitamin D (from dairy products). Diets and supplements that emphasize calcium over magnesium contribute to many magnesium-deficiency problems. High-dairy consumption also adds to this deficiency.

Alan R. Gaby, M.D., gives magnesium supplements to almost every one of his patients. He found that taking extra magnesium eliminated magnesium-deficiency symptoms and prevented calcium deposits like kidney stones and atherosclerosis.

Assessing Your Magnesium Needs

Most doctors suggest you need only the RDA of magnesium (320–420 mg) each day. But magnesium expert Mildred S. Seelig, M.D., disagrees. She says this RDA is based on an erroneous theory and that we need much more. A review on magnesium from the Yale School of Medicine supports Dr. Seelig in its finding that magnesium deficiencies are common. Today, more nutrition-oriented doctors are emphasizing the importance of additional magnesium for their patients.

The theory on which today's RDA is based stated that only half the magnesium we get in our foods and supplements is absorbed. It went on to say that since our kidneys can recirculate magnesium, like they can with calcium, there is no real magnesium deficiency. But since the RDAs were established, follow-up studies indicate that we don't absorb this much magnesium at all. What's more, unabsorbed magnesium is not recirculated, but excreted. Since your kidneys recirculate calcium, this creates an even greater need for additional magnesium.

Your diet and lifestyle may create a need for still more magnesium. A high-salt diet, drinking alcohol, taking hormones, and using diuretic medications all increase the requirement for this mineral, as do tight, painful muscles, heart disease, and osteoporosis.

Some people need equal amounts of magnesium and calcium. Others need even more magnesium than calcium. Since the side effects from taking too much magnesium are mild—loose stools, diarrhea, or stomach irritation—many health practitioners suggest taking it to bowel tolerance. They have their patients add supplemental magnesium up to 1,000 mg a day until they have comfortably loose stools. Some people can tolerate only 100 mg of magnesium a day while others can take as much as 1,000 mg.

Symptoms of Magnesium Deficiency

Constipation is one possible sign of a magnesium deficiency. Increasing magnesium relaxes the intestinal muscles and often alleviates constipation. Before taking magnesium for constipation, check with your doctor to make sure you have no underlying health problem that's causing this condition.

Craving chocolate is another possible sign of a magnesium deficiency, since chocolate contains more magnesium than any other food. When magnesium is increased, chocolate cravings can take a backseat to simply enjoying this flavor. Instead of trying to resist eating chocolate, you might want to increase your magnesium and see if you still crave it as much.

Sore muscles, headaches, tight muscles, irregular heartbeat, PMS, cramps, heart disease, and osteoporosis are other signs that you may need more magnesium. If you're taking a lot of supplemental calcium or eating a diet high in dairy, you may need less calcium, as well.

How Calcium Affects Magnesium Needs

If you're taking a calcium-magnesium supplement, you may not be getting enough magnesium because most supplements contain twice as much calcium as magnesium. In theory, this makes sense because your body contains more calcium than magnesium. But practically speaking, this ratio leaves many people with unabsorbed calcium and a need for more magnesium.

Hypocalcemia
Abnormally low levels of calcium in the blood that can lead to low magnesium and kidney problems.

High calcium, accompanied by low magnesium, can lead to a condition called hypocalcemia. Hypocalcemia, in turn, leads to hypomagnesia, or low magnesium. Correcting both of these imbalances requires an increase in one mineral: magnesium.

Sometimes both calcium and magnesium levels are low. When a person with low calcium and low magnesium is given extra calcium, both levels remain low. When extra magnesium is added, both levels improve. Magnesium is one important key to calcium absorption. Since calcium and magnesium are both absorbed in the same sites in your intestines, too much calcium prevents you from absorbing magnesium.

Foods That Interfere with Magnesium

Magnesium is normally excreted in the urine. Some foods increase this excretion. They include high amounts of alcohol, caffeine, sugars of any kind (even fruits and fruit juices), colas, and animal protein. Some drugs, like diuretics, also increase urinary excretion of magnesium. Other medications, like Digoxin (used for heart problems) and Cisplatin (a chemotherapy drug), block the body's ability to absorb and retain magnesium. In addition, a high-fat diet interferes with the absorption of magnesium. This is because when fats and magnesium are combined, they form soaps that prevent magnesium from being absorbed.

Foods High in Magnesium

Magnesium is found in chlorophyll, which is why green leafy vegetables are a good source of this mineral. For example, one cup of cooked spinach contains more than 100 mg.

Magnesium is stored in the outer layer of grains. You can increase your dietary magnesium simply by eating more whole grains. A cup of wild rice contains 238 mg of magnesium, while a cup of whole-wheat flour has 136 mg. One cup of refined, enriched white flour, on the other hand, has only 34 mg of magnesium.

All beans are a good source of magnesium. Split peas and lentils contain the most: 270 mg per cup. Nuts and seeds are also high in magnesium. One-fourth of a cup of almonds, cashews, or

Brazil nuts will give you between 85 and 95 mg of magnesium.

Unfortunately, few people eat nuts, beans, and whole grains daily. This leaves green vegetables as their major food source of magnesium. It's not likely that anyone can get enough magnesium eating one or two helpings of vegetables a day and only occasional servings of whole wheat bread and beans. In addition, today's foods contain less magnesium than they did in the past. It's becoming almost impossible to meet rising magnesium needs with foods that have less magnesium than ever before.

Why Our Foods Are Low in Magnesium

Foods normally high in magnesium, like green vegetables, can only contain good amounts if the soil they grow in has enough. Unless soil is amended with magnesium, spinach, for example, will contain less magnesium than it should. Magnesium is not found in synthetic fertilizers. Unless soil has been amended naturally, your food may have less magnesium than you think. For this reason, organic foods may contain more magnesium than their conventionally grown counterparts.

Magnesium is one of the nutrients removed from grains when they are refined, and it is not replenished when these foods are "enriched." Whole-wheat flour loses 96 percent of its magnesium when it is refined into white flour.

During the refining process from sugarcane to white sugar, 99 percent of the magnesium it originally contained is lost. And up to 50 percent of the magnesium in vegetables is lost in the water in which it is cooked. For this reason, vegetables that are stir-fried will have more magnesium than those that have been boiled or steamed.

Even the water you drink helps determine how much magnesium you get. Most of our drinking water has been fluoridated. The magnesium naturally found in drinking water is lost during fluoridation. In addition, hard water has more magnesium than soft water. A number of studies have shown that people who drink soft water have more deaths from heart disease than those who drink hard water.

Since fats, meats, and dairy contain very low amounts of magnesium, it's no wonder that we have difficulty getting enough of this important mineral from our food. When dietary sources are not enough, it's time to add magnesium supplements.

Taking Magnesium Supplements

The American Diabetes Association suggests that magnesium chloride is more soluble than most other forms. But there are many well-absorbed forms including magnesium glycinate, magnesium citrate, magnesium aspartate, magnesium gluconate, magnesium lactate, and magnesium amino acid chelate.

The least absorbable forms are magnesium oxide and magnesium hydroxide. They need to be in the presence of stomach acid to be broken down and used. If you're taking antacids or have poor hydrochloric acid (HCl) production due to aging, you may want to avoid these forms of magnesium.

Guy E. Abraham, M.D., who has researched magnesium's role in PMS and osteoporosis, says that any form of magnesium is fine if there's enough hydrochloric acid present. Since your stomach makes HCl to help digest certain foods, it's best to take magnesium supplements along with, or right after, meals.

CONCLUSION

There's no doubt that calcium is an extremely important mineral to help build healthy bones. Our need for this mineral increases throughout our lives at critical times, such as during childhood when bones are forming, and during pregnancy when a fetus needs extra bone-building nutrients. It helps regulate our heart and blood pressure, protects some people against colon cancer, and, if enough can get into our bones, guards against osteoporosis.

But by emphasizing calcium in our diets and supplements, many people have created a magnesium deficiency. This deficiency can affect a wide variety of health conditions from a simple headache to arthritis or a deadly heart attack. It may not be a good idea to take high amounts of calcium supplements, especially when magnesium intake is relatively low. A lower quantity of well-absorbed calcium appears to be more appropriate.

While our need for calcium has remained constant for hundreds of years, our need for magnesium has increased with changes in lifestyle, diet, and the stresses of daily living. Dietary stressors, including too much sugar, alcohol, and caffeine, have left many people deficient in magnesium. This important mineral has been depleted from our soil and removed from foods during refining processes. Yet, as we have seen, without sufficient magnesium, the calcium we require is unable to make its way into bone and other tissues.

The answer is to reduce stress or find ways to handle it better, increase magnesium in our diets and supplements, and evaluate our particular nutritional requirements for calcium. Finally, to be most easily absorbed, these two minerals should come in contact with some form of acid, like the hydrochloric acid naturally secreted by our stomachs.

Calcium and magnesium supplements should be attached to an acid, like citric acid (citrate), aspartic acid (aspartate), or malic acid (malate), for best absorption. When it comes to calcium and magnesium, you are not what you eat. You are what you eat, digest, and absorb.

SELECTED
REFERENCES

Abraham, GE. The calcium controversy. *The Journal of Applied Nutrition*, Fall 1982; 34(2).

Abraham, GE, and Flechas, JD. Management of fibromyalgia: Rationale for the use of magnesium and malic acid. *Journal of Nutritional Medicine*, 1992; 3: 49–59.

Briscoe, AM, and Ragan, C. Effect of magnesium on calcium metabolism in man. *American Journal of Clinical Nutrition*, Nov. 1966.

Brown, SE. Osteoporosis: Sorting fact from fallacy. *The Network News, National Women's Health Network*, July/August 1988.

Bushinsky, DA, Monk, RD. Calcium. *The Lancet*, July 25, 1998; 352: 306–311.

Cumming RG, Cummings SR, et al. Calcium intake and fracture risk: Results from the first study of osteoporotic fractures. *Epidemiology* 1997; 145: 926.

Durlach, J., Ed. First International Symposium on Magnesium Deficiency in Human Pathology, Paris, Springer, Verlag, 1971; 11.

Feskanich, D, Willett, WC, Stampfer, MJ, Colditz, GA. Milk, dietary calcium, and bone fracture risk in women: A 12-year prospective study. *American Journal of Public Health*, 1997; 87 (6): 992–997.

Heaney, RP, Recker, RR, and Weaver, CM. Absorbability of calcium sources: The limited role of solubility. *Calcified Tissue International*, 1990; 46.

Hornyak, M., et al. Magnesium therapy for periodic leg movements-related insomnia and restless legs syndrome: An open pilot study. *Sleep,* Aug. 1, 1998; 21(5).

Hudson, Tori, N.D. *Women's Encyclopedia of Natural Medicine.* Los Angeles: Keats Publishing, 1999.

Levenson, DI, and Bockman, RS. A review of calcium preparations. *Nutrition Reviews,* 1994; 52(7).

Lipkin, M, and Newmark, H. Effect of added dietary calcium on colonic epithelial-cell proliferation in subjects at high risk for familial colonic cancer. *The New England Journal of Medicine,* Nov. 28, 1985; 1381–1384.

McLaren-Howard, J, et al. Hormone replacement therapy and osteoporosis: Bone enzymes and nutrient imbalances. *The Journal of Nutritional and Environmental Medicine,* 1998; 8.

McLean, RM. Magnesium and its therapeutic uses: A review. *The American Journal of Medicine,* Jan. 1994; 96: 63–76.

Riis B, Thomsen K, Christinsen C. Does calcium supplementation prevent postmenopausal bone loss? *The New England Journal of Medicine,* 1987; 316: 173.

Seelig, MS. Interrelationship of magnesium and estrogen in cardiovascular and bone disorders, eclampsia, migraine and premenstrual syndrome. *Journal of the American College of Nutrition,* 1993; 12(4).

Seelig, MS. Adverse stress reactions and magnesium deficiency: preventive and therapeutic implications. *Journal of the American College of Nutrition* 1992; 11:609/Abstract 40.

Teo, K, et al. Effect of intravenous magnesium on mortality in myocardial infarction. *Circulation,* 1990; 82: 111–393.

Weaver, K. Magnesium and its role in vascular reactivity and coagulation. *Contemporary Nutrition,* 1987; 12(3).

OTHER BOOKS
AND RESOURCES

Gaby, Alan R., M.D. *Preventing and Reversing Osteoporosis.* Rocklin, CA: Prima Publishing, 1994.
Solid information on bone health with information on calcium-to-magnesium ratio for women of all ages.

Gittelman, Ann Louise. *Super Nutrition for Menopause.* Garden City Park, NY: Avery Publishing Group, 1998.
A comprehensive program for menopausal and postmenopausal women with guidelines for calcium and magnesium intake.

Kirschmann, Gayla J., and Kirschmann, John D. *Nutrition Almanac,* Fourth Edition. New York: McGraw-Hill, 1996.
Contains charts with vitamin and mineral content of common foods.

Let's Live Magazine
Consumer magazine with emphasis on the health benefits of vitamins, minerals, and herbs.
Customer service:
1-800-676-4333
P.O. Box 74908
Los Angeles, CA 90004
Subscriptions: 12 issues per year, $19.95 in the U.S.; $31.95 outside the U.S.

Physical Magazine

Magazine oriented to body builders and other serious athletes.

Customer service:
1-800-676-4333
P.O. Box 74908
Los Angeles, CA 90004

Subscriptions: 12 issues per year, $19.95 in the U.S.; $31.95 outside the U.S.

The Nutrition Reporter™ newsletter

Monthly newsletter that summarizes recent medical research on vitamins, minerals, and herbs.

Customer service:
P.O. Box 30246
Tucson, AZ 85751-0246
e-mail: jack@thenutritionreporter.com
www.nutritionreporter.com

Subscriptions: $26 per year (12 issues) in the U.S.; $32 U.S. or $48 CNC for Canada; $38 for other countries

Women's Health Letter

Monthly newsletter written by health writer and nutritionist Nan Kathryn Fuchs, Ph.D., with cutting-edge information for women over age fifty.

Soundview Publications
1-800-728-2288
P.O. Box 467939
Atlanta, Georgia 31146-7939

Subscription: 12 issues per year; $39 in the U.S.; $52 outside the U.S.

INDEX

BASIC HEALTH PUBLICATIONS USER'S GUIDES TO NUTRITIONAL SUPPLEMENTS

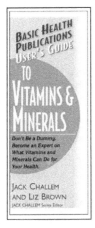

USER'S GUIDE TO VITAMINS & MINERALS

Jack Challem & Liz Brown

Are vitamins really good for you? How about minerals? Thousands of scientific studies say definitely! Vitamins and minerals are required for every aspect of your health—your heart, resistance to infection and cancer, and even for thinking clearly. The *User's Guide to Vitamins & Minerals* explains how these remarkable nutrients can make a big difference in your health.

About the Authors: Jack Challem, a leading American health writer, is editor of *The Nutrition Reporter*™ newsletter (www.nutritionreporter.com) and principal author of *Syndrome X: The Complete Nutrition Program to Prevent and Reverse Insulin Resistance.* His scientific articles have appeared in *Medical Hypotheses, Free Radical Biology and Medicine,* and the *Journal of the National Cancer Institute.* He is also editor for the User's Guide Nutritional Supplements series.

Liz Brown is a freelance health and nutrition writer based in Portland, Oregon. She earned a B.S. in Nutrition from the University of Minnesota-Twin Cities and regularly contributes articles to various magazines and newspapers.

ISBN: 978-1-59120-004-8 • 96 pages
Health/Nutrition

USER'S GUIDE TO WOMEN'S HEALTH SUPPLEMENTS

Laurel Vukovic, MSW

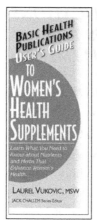

Women have their own distinctive biology and health issues: menstruation, pregnancy, menopause, and breast cancer—to name a few. Many vitamins, minerals, herbal remedies, and medicinal foods can help them to adjust to the changes in their bodies. The Basic Health Publications *User's Guide to Women's Health Supplements* explains how vitamins, minerals, and herbs can help women feel better and stay healthier.

About the Author: Laurel Vukovic, MSW, has been a psychotherapist, herbalist, teacher, and writer for more than two decades. Since 1992, she has been a columnist and contributing editor for *Natural Health* magazine. She is the author of several books, including *Herbal Healing Secrets for Women* and *Journal of Desires.*

ISBN: 978-1-59120-035-2 • 96 pages
Health/Nutrition

For more information about Basic Health Publications User's Guide to Nutritional Supplements Series, or for our catalog, please contact us at the address below.

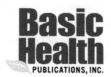

Basic Health
PUBLICATIONS, INC.